Udo Erasmus

Choosing the Right Fats

for
- **Vibrant Health**
- **Weightloss**
- **Energy**
- **Vitality**

alive books

Vancouver
Canada

D0451858

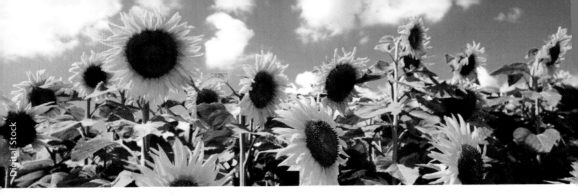

Digital Stock

C o n t e n t s

Note: Conversions in this book (from imperial to metric) are not exact. They have been rounded to the nearest measurement for convenience. Exact measurements are given in imperial. The recipes in this book are by no means to be taken as therapeutic. They simply promote the philosophy of both the author and *alive* books in relation to whole foods, health and nutrition, while incorporating the practical advice given by the author in the first section of the book.

Recipes with Healing Fats

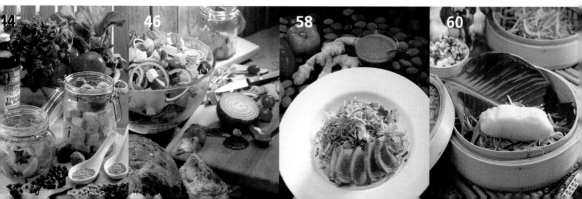

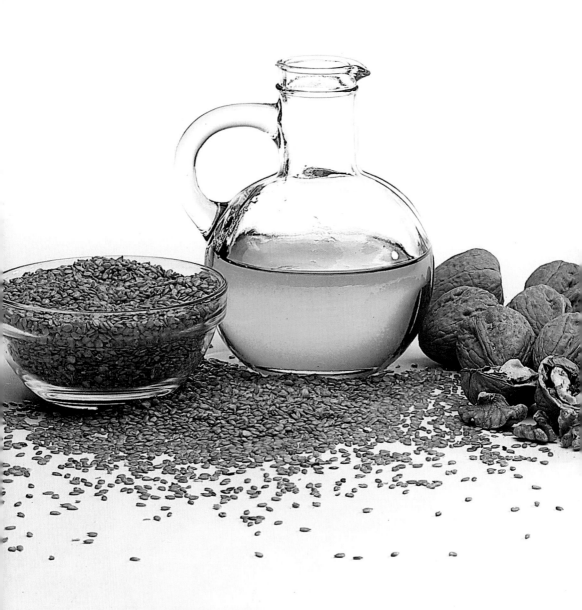

If you were told one of the secrets of good health, would you listen carefully and act accordingly?

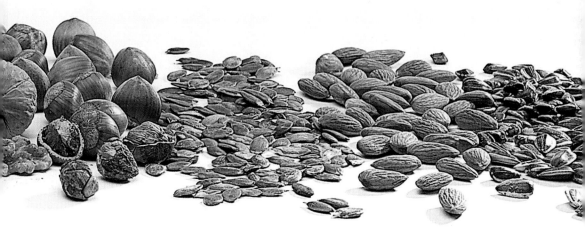

Introduction . . . .

What if someone confided in you one of the great secrets of life and good health? All you had to do was to consume a certain food. This was no ordinary food, but one essential to all people and animals. It was so important that, if not eaten in sufficient amounts, a person became ill, developed symptoms of its deficiency, became progressively sicker and eventually died. But luckily, if caught in time, the secret food could be eaten, and the body healed.

If you were told one of the secrets of life and good health, would you listen carefully and act accordingly? Of course you would. Allow us, then, to introduce you to the essential fats found in healing oils.

Dispel from your mind the negative images conjured up when you read the word fat. Forget the smoky deep fat fryers at your local diner. Forget the sticky oil slick in the bacon pan. Instead contemplate the delicate amber-golden liquid from freshly - pressed nuts and seeds of flax or almonds, the less colorful oils from sunflower, sesame, and hazelnut; and the lively green of pumpkin, pistachio, and extra virgin olive oils.

Each nut and seed contains the germ of a new life and all the food a tiny plant needs to begin growing. But these seeds have life-giving properties for us, too. By extracting the oil from sufficient quantities of seeds we are able to produce oily juices vital to our health in a concentrated form.

Fats that are Essential to Life and Good Health

Plant oils contain ingredients essential to our very survival. They are called essential fatty acids or essential fats, for short, and they feed every part of the body. They provide energy-rich food, or fuel to every cell, tissue, gland, and organ. They are vital to all body structures and many functions. Throughout our lifetime, our brains and nerves, hearts and arteries, reproductive systems, and all cells, tissues, glands, and organs need and use up essential fats.

Because of the dominance of our brain and nervous systems, tissues richest in essential fats, humans have the highest fat requirement of all creatures on the planet. We need at least 15 to 20% of our calories to be essential fat-rich oils. Given the right kinds of fats, this essential fat intake can go as high as 60%. Dr. Michael Crawford, from the UK, suggests that n-3 fatty acids played a key role in increasing the size of the human brain during the course of human evolution.

If this is true, then we can say that fatty acids, found in healing oils, make us human.

Two Essential Fatty Acids: Omega-3 (n-3) and Omega-6 (n-6)

Of less than fifty essential nutrients that by definition we must have and cannot live without, two come from fats and oils. They are known as essential fatty acids or essential fats.

N-3 or Alpha-Linolenic Acid

The essential fat most likely to be in short supply in our modern diet is n-3 or alpha-linolenic acid. In nature, small amounts of it are found in dark green vegetables, but flax is our richest source. High fat, cold water fish like salmon, sardines, mackerel, albacore (white) tuna, and rainbow trout contain derivatives of the n-3, such as eicosapentaenoic acid (EPA) used for hormone (eicosanoid) production, and doxosahexaenoic acid (DHA) required for brain development, brain function, and vision.

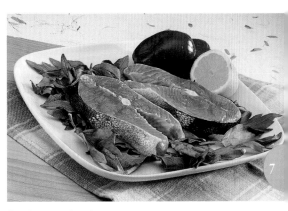

Salmon is a good food source of a derivative of n-3.

N-6 or Linoleic Acid

The other essential fat is n-6 or linoleic acid. It is found in most seeds and nuts. Small amounts are found in grains and vegetables. In temperate climates, n-6 fats are far more abundant than n-3 fats. Fish, dairy, eggs, and meat contain the n-6 derivative arachidonic acid (AA), which is required both for hormone (eicosanoid) production and brain function.

Both essential fats are sensitive to destruction by light, oxygen, or air, and high temperature. This is why they are damaged and become toxic when we fry them. But the n-3 essential fat is five times more chemically sensitive, and therefore five times more quickly destroyed than the n-6 fat.

Unlike other essential nutrients, which can be dried, powdered, and stored with little deterioration, products rich in essential fats must be made with great care. They should be packaged in dark glass, refrigerated or frozen, and used with care in order to retain their health-promoting and health-maintaining functions. Oil shrinks when frozen, so glass bottles are fine for storage.

When both essential fats are consumed in the right amounts and ratios to one another, the body makes several derivatives with important functions. From three of the derivatives (one from the n-3 and two from the n-6), it makes hormones called eicosanoids or prostaglandins. These regulate what goes on in every tissue in the body, all the time.

You may be familiar with some hormones. Insulin is a protein, and thyroid hormone is made from an amino acid. Hormones such as: estrogen, testosterone, and cortisone are made from cholesterol.

But much less well known are the eicosanoid hormones, which can be made only from the healing essential fats.

Fats have other names . . .
Fat (hard at room temperature) = Oil (liquid at room temperature) = Lipid (includes both hard and liquid).

Healing Fats by other names . . . . .
The ingredients from fats that are essential to our life (omega 3 and omega 6 essential fatty acids) go by many names. These names include:
Healing fat = good fat = good oil = right fat = right oil = essential fat = healing oil = essential fatty acid. We use these terms interchangeably, but they all mean the same thing. These are substances found in fats, which the body can't make but needs for health, and must therefore obtain from foods.

Note: The term essential oil refers to fragrance (or essence) oils found in plants, e.g. cedar, lavender, peppermint, patchouli, and so on. Essential oils are completely different from essential fats that we are talking about, because essence oils are not essential to human life.

Healing Fats by family nicknames . . . .
Healing fats, members of two families called omega 3 and omega 6, have several nicknames.

Omega 3 = alpha-linolenic acid = LNA = ALA = w3 = w-3 = n3 = n-3. At the beginning of a sentence, n-3 becomes N-3.

Omega 6 = linoleic acid = LA = w6 = w-6 = n6 = n-6. At the beginning of a sentence, n-6 becomes N-6.

Most experts in fats now use the n-3 and n-6 abbreviations for the two classes of healing fats, so these most common abbreviations for healing essential fats are also used in the book.

You can find more information on the healing fats in *Fats That Heal, Fats That Kill*, available through alive Books.

The primary building blocks of health are called essential nutrients. The word essential, used in the context of nutrition, has a precise, specific meaning.

1. An essential nutrient is a substance the body must have in order to live and function normally. The body cannot manufacture any essential nutrient from other substances, and must therefore get it from the outside environment in the form of foods or supplements.
2. If the body obtains too little of an essential nutrient, deficiency symptoms develop and a person's health deteriorates. Symptoms of essential nutrient deficiencies, degenerative in nature, progressively worsen in time. And, if the deficiency remains uncorrected, the person eventually dies. Simply stated - we cannot live without essential nutrients.
3. Degenerative symptoms can be reversed and health restored by returning the missing essential nutrient to the diet.
4. A nutrient is only called essential once researchers have identified at least one biochemical reaction that requires the presence of the nutrient, and without which that biochemical reaction could not take place.

Essential Nutrients include:

for adults:	• 20 minerals
	• 13 vitamins
for children:	• 8 essential amino acids (derived from proteins); 2 additional amino acids are essential, and one further amino acid is essential for premature infants.
	• Included in the essential nutrients are 2 essential fatty acids, which come from fats and oils

Healing Fats and the Human Diet . . . .

Fat in a Traditional Diet

Most traditional diets that kept people free of degenerative conditions derived 15% or more of the calories from fats. The tradition-

9

al diet of the Inuit included up to 60% of calories from raw whale blubber, seal fat, and fish. In spite of this super fat-rich diet, they were free of blood clot-induced heart attacks and strokes. They were free of cancer, diabetes, and multiple sclerosis. Their high mortality was unrelated to fats. They lived in a harsh Arctic climate where greens were scarce and their burst blood vessel strokes were mostly due to a lack of vitamin C. The Inuit also suffered vitamin E deficiencies because cold water fish do not require it, and so the Inuit had almost none of this antioxidant vitamin in their mostly meat and fish diet. Osteoporosis in the Inuit resulted from a high protein intake, which removes minerals from the body.

The traditional Inuit diet was rich in essential n-3 and n-6. In contrast the diets of people in affluent Western countries today are low in the protective n-3: n-6 at a ratio of 1-10 or even 1-20; n-3 intake is less than 20% of levels eaten by people in the year 1850. Western diets have been destructively processed, producing toxic molecules. In addition the ratio of 3 to 6 is wrong, too many of the fats we eat are too rich in saturated fats and twisted trans- fats.

Recommended Percentage of Fats in Daily Calories

The following advice applies to healing fats produced and stored with care and consumed in the proper ratio of n-3 to n-6 .

Take as much essential fat as is required to make your skin soft and velvety, which amounts to about 1 tablespoon (15ml) per 50 pounds (22kg) of body weight per day in cold weather, and less than that in warm weather. 2 to 5 tablespoons (30 to 75ml) per day are optimal for adults. Up to 10 tablespoons (150ml) per day (about 50% of calories) can be used to lose weight, speed healing, build muscles, and help reverse degenerative conditions caused by getting too little essential fat.

Striking a Balance: the Right Ratio of N-3 to N-6

Researchers have not agreed on the best ratio of n-3 to n-6. Some have suggested that the perfect ratio is one part n-3 to every four or five parts n-6. They base their opinion on enzyme studies of tissue cultures, and the fact that n-3 are converted four or five times faster than n-6.

Some people suggest that the historical ratio was 1:1. The ratio in traditional diets varied with latitude and with seasonal and climatic fluctuations. The higher the latitude into Arctic and Antarctic, the higher the n-3 content of the diet. The closer to the tropics, the lower the amount of n-3 and n-6 in the traditional diet. A 1:1 ratio was impossible to achieve in many parts of the world, due to variations in environment, based on climate.

The traditional Inuit ratio was 2.5: 1….and did not produce n-6 deficiency symptoms. The traditional Mediterranean diets was about 1: 4….and did not produce n-3 deficiency symptoms.

The brains of both Inuit and Italians contain a ratio of 1: 1, indicating that the body's tissues and organs take what they need from whatever food sources are provided. Radically different diets can both provide adequate essential fats. The key requirement is that the food supply includes adequate amounts of the right quality, and enough of both healing fats.

Healthy people can consume foods with a wide range of ratios (2.5: 1 to 1: 6). Sick people respond to n-3 enrichment in more than twice as many conditions as n-6 enrichment.

In practice, I have consistently seen that a ratio richer in n-3 produces better therapeutic results for most people. From 15 years of experience working with oils, I have developed what I call a practical ratio, a ratio that consistently gives the best results. I have found that the exclusive use of flax (linseed) oil, rich in n-3, but low in n-6 (3.5-4: 1) can lead to problems such as dry eyes, skipped heart beat, painful finger joints, and fragile, thin skin. It can also lead to eczema-like skin problems, and to lowered immune function. This is because essential fats compete for enzyme space in our cells, and the overabundance of n-3 in flax crowds out the n-6, leading to n-6 deficiency.

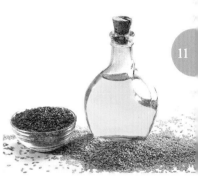

Flax oil is particularly rich in n-3 essential fats but too low in n-6.

No traditional diet has the high ratio of flax oil. The Inuit diet, with a ratio of 2.5: 1, is the n-3-richest traditional diet that does not lead to n-6 deficiency. Yes, there can be too much of a good thing. Be sure you get the right ratio of n-3 to n-6 for long-term best effects.

The best ratio of essential fats is obtained by blending several healing oils. After much experimentation I have come up with a blend I call Udo's Choice Oil Blend, packaged in amber glass and enclosed in a box to protect it from all light.

I have found that a ratio of about 2: 1, a ratio almost as rich in n-3, as that of the traditional Inuit, works best.

Your intake of n-3 is likely to have decreased to ⅙ of what people consumed in 1850. N-3 deficiency is widespread. This is due to the fact that n-3 is very sensitive to destruction during processing, and is removed from foods to extend product shelf life.

A dificiency in n-3 is more difficult to indentify than a n-6. The reason is that n-6 can partially cover n-3 deficiencies. N-3, on the other hand, cannot cover for a shortage of n-6. If your body suffers an n-3 deficiency, you may have the following symptoms.

- Retarded growth
- Behavioral change
- Weakness
- Weakened vision
- Learning problems
- Depression
- Hyperactivity, attention deficit, and dyslexia
- Poor motor coordination
- Poor muscle growth
- Impaired healing of injuries
- Tingling sensations in arms and legs
- Insulin resistance
- High triglycerides
- High blood pressure
- Sticky platelets, or tendency to form clots in arteries, leading to heart attack, stroke, or embolism
- High lipoprotein(a) - a strong predictive risk factor for cardiovascular disease
- High fibrinogen a clotting risk factor
- Inflammation in tissues
- Leaky gut
- Allergies
- Auto-immune conditions
- Increased susceptibility to tumor growth
- Water retention or edema
- Dry or inflamed skin
- Low metabolic rate
- Low energy level
- Lowered thyroid and adrenal function
- Low testosterone level

N-6 Deficiency Symptoms

- Eczema-like skin eruptions
- Hair loss
- Water loss through the skin, with attendant thirst; common in diabetes insipidus, and often seen in hyperactive children
- Behavioral changes
- Fatty infiltration of the liver
- Kidney malfunction
- Drying up of glands
- Susceptibility to infection
- Failure of wounds to heal
- Sterility in males
- Miscarriage in females
- Arthritis-like conditions
- Heartbeat abnormalities that can lead to cardiac arrest
- Growth retardation
- Dry skin and hair
- Brittle nails
- Dry eyes
- Elevated cholesterol

Udo's Choice Oil Blend Combines Healing Oils and More

Udo's Choice Oil Blend includes three high quality, organic, unrefined oils and seven other vital ingredients. Each was chosen for its specific health-promoting properties. Organic flax oil supplies n-3 fatty acids. Organic sunflower and sesame oils provide n-6 fatty acids. Unrefined evening primrose seed oil supplies n-6 and its derivative GLA. These four, and rice germ and oat germ oils were selected over many other oils because they are rich in natural, oil-soluble phytonutrients with powerful healing benefits. Some of these oils are not commercially available in unrefined form, so innovation in production had to be developed.

In addition to the six oils, Udo's Choice Oil Blend contains medium chain triglycerides (or MCTs), found in coconut oil. These are easy for the liver to metabolize and have strong anti-viral, anti-fungal, and anti-bacterial properties. MCTs lower cho-

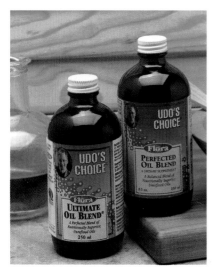

lesterol, improve fat absorption (which in the case of the essential fats is desirable), and have tumor-inhibiting effects. And, they also taste good!

The blend also contains GMO-free lecithin and natural phytosterols. Our cell membranes and the skins of HDL and LDL cholesterol are made from lecithin. Phytosterols block cholesterol absorption and can lower high cholesterol by up to 25%. They also enhance immune function and protect the prostate gland.

Oil-soluble free radical scavengers Vitamin E and tocotrienols are added to preserve freshness.

Why I developed the Oil Blend and Became Known as the "Fat Man"
Until 1987, most oil in North American supermarkets had been manufactured with shelf life rather than consumer health in mind. To last a long time without spoiling on a grocer's shelf, good oil was processed to the point where it was damaged. Some substances were removed, and some molecules were changed from natural and health supporting to unnatural and toxic. I decided to see if I could do better. I developed methods for making oils with human health in mind.

The first oil I developed was flax oil and I packaged it in black plastic. In 1993, I learned that estrogen mimickers leach from some plastics into the environment and change reproductive structures and reproductive behaviors in animals. I changed my mind about using plastic to package oils and other liquids, because I concluded that we know too little about the possible effects of plastics on health and the environment to take a chance. I changed to amber glass bottles.

Committed to using flax oil, I personally discovered that using this oil exclusively created symptoms of n-6 deficiency such as: dry eyes, arthritic-like finger joints, thin papery skin, and - most frightening - skipped heart beats.

In 1994, I replaced flax oil with a blend of oils with a better ratio of n-3 to n-6 healing essential fats. I packaged it in amber glass, put the glass bottle into a box to protect it from light, and stored the oil blend in the refrigerator or freezer. I began marketing the oil blend through health food stores and practitioners.

I have traveled in North America, Europe, and Australia, telling the story of fats that kill and fats that heal. I have given thousands of presentations and interviews.

Since 1987, I have also worked to improve the health of animals through improved fat nutrition.

The Healing Properties of Phytonutrients

Besides essential fats, other oil-soluble substances are present in oils pressed with care from seeds and nuts, and not subjected to any additional processing. In such oils, phytonutrients make up about 2% of the oil, and they have major health benefits.

They go by several names. Commercial oil processors who want a chemically pure, fully refined and deodorized, long shelf life supermarket oil call them impurities and remove them. People interested in health call them phytonutrients or 'minor' ingredients. These plant-based, natural, nutritional molecules are some of nature's best medicines. They are abundant in the membranes of green foods, herbs, seeds, and nuts.

The oil-soluble phytonutrients found in oils contrast with better known water-soluble phytonutrients such as: bioflavonoids, proanthocyanidin pigments, and plant-based antioxidants. Phytonutrients are called nutraceuticals by the pharmaceutical industry. Sometimes they are called phytochemicals. Because of their many benefits, the drug industry now wants to be seen to have invented and to own them. But they are natural plant constituents, not drugs.

Refined Oil is not a Healing Oil

During refining processes, most phytonutrients have been partially removed or destroyed from common supermarket and other oils. These processes include degumming, refining, bleaching, and deodorizing. They are used to produce uniformly colorless, odorless, and tasteless products. What is gained in extended shelf life is lost in health benefits. If the label does not say, "unrefined", then the oil has been processed. The exception is extra virgin (but not 'extra light' or '100%) olive oil. Extra virgin olive oil has not been processed and is unrefined, even if the label does not state it.

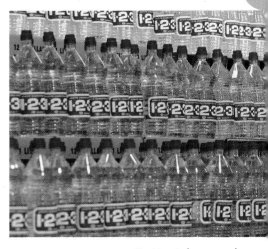

Heat treated, processed oils are <u>not</u> healthy oils the keyword to look for is "unrefined oils"

Healing oils should be pressed from organically-grown seeds and nuts. They are best stored in brown glass, and refrigerated. You will find them most often marketed in health food stores and websites.

Some phytonutrients lower the body's cholesterol level. Others improve digestion, and liver and gall bladder functions. Some have anti-oxidant functions. Some protect the cardiovascular system. Some have specific benefits for inner organs.

Phytonutrients include a wide range of different molecules with therapeutic benefits. Best known are cholesterol lowering phytosterols; magnesium-rich and detoxifying chlorophyll; and protective antioxidants like carotene, vitamin E (or tocopherols), and polyphenols. But there are hundreds of others that are not yet household words.

Healing Oils and the Complex Balance of Energy, Weight and Diet . . . .

Essential Fats and Energy

Essential fats have many vital functions, but one of their really interesting features is that they improve energy levels. Think of them (especially n-3) as super-fuel for your body. They promote high energy and stamina in several ways.

First, they make red blood cell membranes more flexible and the inside of the arteries more slippery, so that red blood cells slide through capillaries more easily. This means that delivery of nutrients and oxygen to tissues occurs more effectively. Since energy is produced by the interaction of oxygen with nutrients, better delivery of these to tissues means more energy.

Second, they optimize the production of the oxygen-carrying red pigment hemoglobin. This brings about better delivery of oxygen to tissues. Oxygen is necessary for most of the reactions by which energy is made available for tissue functions.

Third, essential fats optimize thyroid, adrenal, and other glandular functions. Optimum gland function leads to optimum energy production throughout the body.

Fourth, essential fats up-regulate the expression of many of the genes that code for enzymes involved in energy production, fat burning, and heat production (thermogenesis).

Finally, essential fats may increase energy by helping the body obtain more oxygen when more oxygen is needed. They can also increase oxygen metabolism, and thereby increase oxidation rate, increase metabolic rate, increase energy levels, and increase stamina. That means it will take longer to get tired from exertion. Essential fats also speed recovery, shortening the time it takes fatigued muscles to get their energy back. Essential fats also speed the healing of injuries.

How fats increase energy is a complex matter, but we know for sure that essential fats do increase energy. N-3 does it best. Energy increase is most apparent in athletes, the elderly, and those suffering from degenerative conditions. But it can also be observed in overweight persons, middle-aged, and even in young people.

When I first started adding healing oils to my diet I noticed a dramatic increase in my energy level. Instead of getting tired at 11:00 p.m., I would find myself still working at 2:00 or 3:00 a.m. I did not experience a coffee-like buzz; just that the energy was there when I needed it. I slept better, needed about an hour less sleep, and woke up more refreshed.

In 1988, a professional trainer increased the intake of n-3 in football players. He found that they could chase the ball longer, recovered more quickly from fatigue and that their injuries healed in one third to one half of the usual time.

Since then I have recommended incorporating healing oils into the diets of athletes in all kinds of sports such as: hockey, baseball, tennis, and soccer and for runners, cyclists, biathletes, tri-athletes, bobsledders, skaters, boxers, martial artists, bodybuilders and weight lifters. One small bodybuilder I met in Miami reported that he increased weight training repetitions within three days of starting 3 tablespoons (45ml) daily of the oil blend. A large bodybuilder in Denmark used 8 tablespoons (120ml) daily with

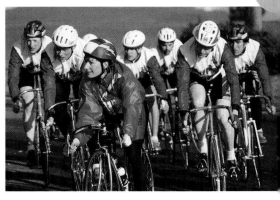

Optimizing essential fats intake improves performance of athletes.

similar effects. Consistently, athletes who push the limits of performance, both in strength and in endurance sports, find that optimizing essential fat intake, and getting n-3 and n-6 in the right ratio, improves their performance. They also recover more rapidly from fatigue caused by lactic acid buildup.

Older people who begin to take fresh, healing oils report that they tire less easily, recover faster, don't get tired as early in the evening, and feel more capable of engaging in physical activity. I know one couple who took up canoeing again in their 70's after giving it up in their 50's for lack of energy.

In another case, an 84-year old woman, bedridden, on 24-hour-a-day care, became virtually self-sufficient within 2 months of getting the essential fats that were lacking in her diet.

Right Fats for the Right Body
By T'ai Erasmus, ISSA

Over the past ten years, essential fatty acids have been an integral part of every individualized sports nutrition meal plan I have developed. Clients from all walks of life, including movie and music celebrities, stunt performers, professional athletes, bodybuilders and fitness competitors consume EFAs as part of their daily ritual. The transformations and feedback have been amazing!

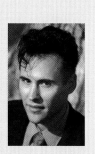

The first reports I receive from clients are noticeable improvements in energy levels, followed by a reduction in body fat. They observe either how they look in the mirror or how their clothes fit. Finally, they note that their results are permanent providing they stay consistent with their improved eating habits. All lead to elevated excitement about exercise, nutrition and health.

During my studies of fitness and nutrition, I was taught you should lose no more than one half to one pound of fat per week. That adds up to two to four pounds per month. It doesn't sound like much and many people find it discouraging.

In fact, my personal experience has been different. On average, clients lose anywhere from five to fifteen pounds per month, and it's not muscle. Sound too good to be true? These finding were confirmed by body composition assessments. No fiction, just the facts.

So, how do you do it?
1. Accept that there are no quick fixes.
2. Understand that when you provide your body with the right fuel sources - macronutrients and micronutrients - in the appropriate amounts, your body will look and feel the way you want it to.
3. Make a commitment to accomplish your goals in the healthiest, most effective manner.
4. Stay active.
5. Celebrate your daily accomplishments.
6. Find someone who is qualified to help you organize your plan for success.

Nutrition must be an integral component of his personal training, health and fitness programs. T'ai can be contacted by **e-mail** at **tai@taierasmus.com**.

Essential Fats and Weight

Essential fats can help you normalize your weight and reduce body fat. They will increase your metabolic rate, heat production, and energy levels, which means that you burn more calories, even at rest. They also make you feel more like being physically active, which results in additional calorie burning.

Essential fats play several other roles in weight management. They help your kidneys dump excess water held in your tissues - water that constitutes extra weight. They release water held in tissues swollen by inflammation, which can then be removed from the body. One woman in Norway lost 11 pounds (5 kg) in 7 days using 10 tablespoons (150 ml) of oil blend. There are reports of people losing 120 pounds in 6 weeks. A word of caution: This weight loss must be attributed to water loss. Excess fat cannot be lost so quickly.

Essential fats suppress appetite. They help decrease cravings for junk foods, starches, and sweets. These cravings are often the result of not getting the nutrients you need from the foods you eat. Obtaining the missing essential fats satisfies the craving.

Essential fats also help in weight normalization by elevating mood and lifting depression, removing one major reason why some people overeat. Elevated mood also makes you feel like being more active.

Most interesting, they increase the activity of several genes that make enzymes for fat burning and thermogenesis, and decrease the activity of several other genes that make enzymes for fat production. In other words, they make it harder to make fat and easier to burn fat. N-3 does it best. N-6 does it slightly. The non-essential n-9 (monounsaturated), saturated, and trans- fatty acids do not help the function of these genes at all.

Counting calories

Here's an interesting proposition. Don't count the nine calories per gram in healing oils. Count only sugars and starches, which can be used only for fuel, and saturated & monounsaturated (non-essential fats).

The essential fats are different. Your body does not burn them primarily for energy, but uses them to make membranes, essential fat derivatives with health benefits, and hormones. In addition, essential fat, especially n-3 increases fat and calorie burning. Essential fats, therefore, are fats that keep you slim! I recommend subtracting three calories from the total calorie count for each gram of n-3 in the diet, rather than adding nine. Sounds strange, but that's how it works.

Let me give you another strange-sounding, but true, example. When bodybuilders get ready for competition, they want to get rid of the fat under their skin. They want the muscle fibers to show through the skin. It's called being shredded, and gets them extra marks. To get rid of the skin fat, some builders take up to 14 tablespoons (210 ml) of oil blend daily for two weeks before competition. These fats get rid of fats! Previously, bodybuilders used dangerous diuretics and some died from their use. Now they can safely use the oil blend. In addition, they keep sodium and carbohydrate intake low, and eat more greens and protein.

Fats do not make you Fat

Our society has developed a fat phobia, but it is unfounded. Fats do not make you fat. Surprised? Research shows that in the past 20 years, people in America have reduced their fat intake from 42% of total calories to 33%. This change has come about in response to major ad campaigns by government and interest groups. In the same twenty years, the percentage of the population defined as overweight increased from 25% to 55%. If you're eating less fat, but are getting fatter, it's because you've been misinformed.

There's proof that fats do not make you fat. High fat, high protein diets have been used since the turn of the century for weight management. They work. Unfortunately, such diets often contain bad fats that may cause problems for the liver and kidneys and increase the risk of cancer and cardiovascular disease.

Obesity (more than 30% above ideal body weight) increased from 12% to 17% between 1991 and 1997, at the height of fat phobia. As fat intake decreases, body fat increases. In other words, not eating fats can make you gain body fat.

The commonly held belief that dietary fats cause obesity, and that fat avoidance will keep us slim, is wrong. Fats help to keep you lean. Even better, the essential fats keep you both lean and healthy.

If Fats don't make you Fat, then what does?

It has been known since the turn of the last century and, frankly, back to the time of Hippocrates (500 BC) that diets high in protein and fat, and low in carbohydrates help people reduce body fat. They work because fats suppress appetite.

If you shun fats because you are afraid of getting fat, you end up being hungry all the time, and nibbling on starchy and sweet foods. You end up eating more carbohydrates than your body

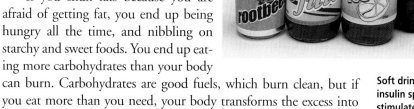

can burn. Carbohydrates are good fuels, which burn clean, but if you eat more than you need, your body transforms the excess into fat and stores it for later. Then you're wearing the excess fuel, waiting for a famine.

Soft drinks set off an insulin spike and stimulate fat production

The worst carbohydrates are white sugar, honey and syrups, added to soft drinks, tea, coffee, sports drinks, juices, candies, cakes, cookies. The sugars these products contain are absorbed very rapidly, set off an insulin spike, and stimulate fat production and the changes that lead to diabetes.

Favourite carbohydrates that cause weight problems include the following: white bread, muffins, potatoes, fries, sweet potatoes, yams, corn, pumpkins, bananas, boxed cereals, pasta, crackers, potato chips, other snacks and convenience foods, other sugar-based sweeteners, and hidden sugar in all kinds of prepared commercial foods like ketchup, bread, and sauces.

All starches and the products made with them will make you fat if you don't burn all that you consume. The more active you are, the more starch you can burn (and therefore eat). The less active you are, the more important it becomes to limit your carbohydrate intake. Each calorie not burned must be turned into fat in the body. That is the body's law: If you don't burn 'em, you wear 'em.

Carbohydrates also increase tissue swelling and water retention. That water, along with the excess fat, makes you heavier and rounder.

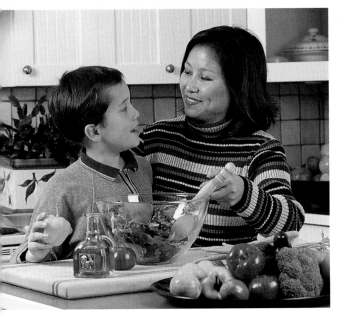

Green vegetables are the most important food group because they are rich in nutrients and low in calories.

Aim for a Healthy Weight Normalization Diet

A healthy weight normalization diet looks exactly the same as a program for optimum health. The most important food group includes the green vegetables, because they are the nutrient-richest and calorie-poorest foods. Also included are the healing fats and proteins, which supply essential nutrients your body cannot produce. If digesting proteins is a problem, I recommend taking digestive enzyme supplements, rich in protein-digesting proteases, with the foods you eat.

Sugars cause many problems because of their fast absorption, and starches must be restricted to the amount actually needed and therefore burned for energy. This is especially important for people with diabetes, blood sugar problems, sedentary people, and those who are overweight. Are you one of these? If so, take heed. Also go easy on fruits, because they contain quite a lot of sugar, and can get you high triglycerides and insulin resistance.

The best sources of carbohydrates include greens such as lettuce, celery, broccoli, spinach, kale, green beans, bok choi, mustard greens, arugula, dandelion greens, green peppers, okra, peas and pea leaves, green weeds and herbs. You can also include other fiber-rich, starch-poor vegetables such as cauliflower and bell peppers.

How do you know how many carbohydrates are too many? If you're putting on weight, you need to eat fewer. An athlete can eat and burn a lot more carbohydrates than a person with a sedentary lifestyle.

Popular Fat Diets Simply Don't Work

Popular high fat diets that typically start the day with bacon and eggs do not work for health. They can contribute to health problems such as cardiovascular disease, high cholesterol, cancer, multiple sclerosis, high blood pressure, and other degenerative diseases. You need more greens and more healing fats than such a diet provides.

A no fat diet is a really bad joke. It will kill anyone who stays on it long enough, because a no fat diet lacks the essential fats, essential nutrients available only through diet. Don't go on a no fat diet. If you're on one, get off right now.

Fake fat diets are relatively new. They contain synthetic substances that have the feel and taste of fat, but are not digested. Through substitution such diets may eliminate some unhealthy fats, but cannot make up for the lost essential fatty acids. They also transport health-supporting oil-soluble nutrients such as carotene, vitamins A, D, K, and E, and phytonutrients, out of the body. Don't waste your money on fake fats. Instead, get the nutritious foods your body needs.

Fat blockers and removers prevent fats from being absorbed. The ads promise that you can eat all the fats you want, as they will be eliminated. Unfortunately blockers cannot differentiate between healthy and unhealthy fats, and remove both the bad and the good fats from the body with the same enthusiasm. If you insist on using these (really quite stupid) fat removers, make sure that you take them at a time set apart from when you eat the necessary healing oils.

Low fat diets deprive us of the fats that heal. They can lead to dry skin; low energy levels; hair loss, high triglycerides; proneness to inflammatory and auto-immune conditions; likelihood of developing leaky gut and allergies; poorer immune function; compromised liver, kidney, gland, and organ functions; increased glucose sensitivity and insulin resistance; reproductive failure; poor growth; mood and behavior changes; and lower testosterone production.

The Right Fat Diet for Health and Weight Management

It's worth repeating: You do not need a high fat, no fat, fake fat, fat remover, or low fat diet. What you need, for the sake of your health, is the right fat diet - a diet that provides optimum amounts of healing fats.

Testimonials of Athetes who added Udo's Choice Oil Blend to their Training programs (15 mL/50 Lb of body weight/day)

Name	Sport	Testimonials
Female, top-level amateur, age 24	Basketball	This athlete experienced much faster recuperation after training sessions. Before entering the trial, she would be dead tired after practice and aching and sore for about an hour. Now she feels as if she can do another training session again in 20-30 minutes.
Male, formerly a participant in strong man contests, won the Danish and Nordic bodybuilding championships in 2001, age, 40's	Body-building	Madsen felt an improvement in his joints. After a few weeks of using the oil, they stopped aching, both during weight-resistance training (5-6 times a week) and afterwards. His skin got better. He felt as if the "lotion was applied from the inside - out." He no longer needed body lotion most of the time despite taking several showers a day.
Male, age, 20's	Body-building	When he started taking oil, Laursen had reached a plateau in his muscular development. He'd been training for nine years, but it seemed as if he couldn't develop his muscle mass any further. After taking the oil, his muscle mass started developing again. His weight has increased by another 15 kg since then. Also, his hair grows much faster and is thicker.
Male, age 24	Boxing	After a few weeks on the trial, his acne and other skin problems cleared up. "All of a sudden, I found myself training 30 minutes or an hour longer than usual, without noticing it."
Male, age 33	Boxing	His concentration improved, making his movements sharper and better defined while boxing. "I ran faster and longer."
Male, type I diabetic, smoker	Boxing	Eriksen experienced improvements in endurance, training intensity, energy level and quickness of recovery after exercise. After a few days of supplementation, it took him only thirty minutes to fall into a deep sleep, as opposed to the one or more hours it previously took him to fall into an uneasy sleep. Also, he dreamt more and could remember his dreams upon waking up in the morning.
Male, type II diabetic, smoker, age 54	Boxing	At one point, he had a short break from the oil, for a few days. He experienced a regression in terms of the positive effects he had felt from the oil such as: increased energy level, and improved stamina and concentration. A few days after starting supplementation with the oil again, things were back to normal.
Male , type II diabetic, age 51	Boxing	This athlete felt stronger and more focused mentally. He felt his thinking was "sharper" and also that he was not stressed as easily. His knees improved. The slight arthritis he had in his right knee, as a result of an operation in 1969, disappeared after a few weeks of oil supplementation.
Male, age 34	Cycling	This cyclist rides between 80 and 100 km a day, as opposed to 50 to 60 km before starting on the oil. His stamina has improved so that he can go longer before getting tired. He reports that he was bothered by continuous sitting sores, which never healed completely. Now they heal quicker and actually disappear completely from time to time.
Female, mountain biking, long distance running, adventure sports, and ashtanga yoga (about 20 hours of practice a week), age 23	Duathlon and Triathlon	A regular oil consumer, Svendsen always recovers in the morning, no matter how much training or hard a competition she has been through. On the few occasions she has gone without the oil for a few days she has felt a regression in terms of how fast she can recuperate from exercise. She was able to complete and win a half-marathon on a tablespoon of oil and a few tablespoons of boiled whole spelt grains which provided her with enough energy. " I wouldn't be able to do without the oil on my present training schedule."
Male, age 37	Duathlon and Triathlon	"The first time I really noticed a difference was when I started training really hard. After three or four weeks of using the oil, I felt things getting better, day to day. I used to get tired as the day progressed and couldn't get my pulse up and going. But with the oil I have lots of energy and keep on training the whole day."
Male, age 50	Weight training	This weight trainer experienced improvements to his chronically painful left shoulder and knee. The left shoulder joint had been damaged in an accident and needed surgery; his knees were stressed from an accident. Before entering the study they bothered him quite a lot and were a limiting factor in terms of training. He wasn't able to train more than twice a week and they kept him awake at night. After the eight weeks of the trial, his joints felt fine within 24 to 48 hours after a workout.

The Cardiovascular System: The Right Fats Lower Blood Fats.

The cardiovascular system requires essential fatty acids for cholesterol transport. The n-3 essential fat lowers high triglycerides (blood fats) very effectively, by up to 65%, which is better than any drug sold for lowering them. This means that the right fats actually *lower* blood fats. If n-3 and n-6 essential fats are consumed in the right ratio (2: 1, n-3: n-6), the body uses them to produce beneficial kinds of hormone-like eicosanoids (prostaglandins). These make platelets less sticky, and decrease the likelihood that a clot will form in an artery to the heart, brain, or other organ.

Healing oils help to lower high blood pressure by relaxing arterial muscle tone. They protect people from heart attacks, strokes, and emboli. They help the kidneys dump excess water and decrease inflammation, which also increases risk of cardiovascular disease. They can lower the levels of a blood-clotting factor (fibrinogen) when that factor is too high. They lower excessively high levels of lipoprotein(a), a very strong risk factor for heart and artery disease. They keep the heartbeat regular; preventing heart beat abnormalities that could lead to cardiac arrest. They also increase the good HDL cholesterol and the HDL: LDL ratio.

If the n-3: n-6 ratio is wrong (the more excessive n-6 intake, the worse the problem gets), the body

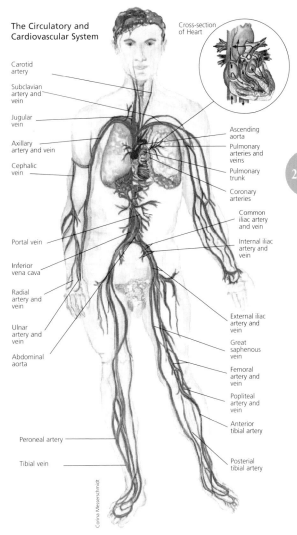

The Circulatory and Cardiovascular System

Cross-section of Heart

Carotid artery
Subclavian artery and vein
Jugular vein
Axillary artery and vein
Cephalic vein
Portal vein
Inferior vena cava
Radial artery and vein
Ulnar artery and vein
Abdominal aorta
Peroneal artery
Tibial vein

Ascending aorta
Pulmonary arteries and veins
Pulmonary trunk
Coronary arteries
Common iliac artery and vein
Internal iliac artery and vein
External iliac artery and vein
Great saphenous vein
Femoral artery and vein
Popliteal artery and vein
Anterior tibial artery
Posterial tibial artery

Corina Messerschmidt

25

can make prostaglandins in a detrimental ratio, which can make platelets more sticky, raise blood pressure, retain water, and increase inflammation. The n-3: n-6 ratio is vitally important. Pay attention to this ratio. It is important for health and long life.

Reducing Cholesterol through Healing Oils and other Products

Healing oils lower cholesterol only slightly on their own but the natural phytosterols found in organic, unrefined healing oils block cholesterol absorption and reabsorption from the gut. They can lower cholesterol by up to 25%. The oil blend I developed is very rich in these good phytosterols. It contains 65mg per 15ml (tablespoon) of oil.

There are other products to lower cholesterol quite reliably. One is a water-soluble fiber called mucilage, which escorts toxins, heavy metals, and cholesterol out of the body, as well as stabilizes blood glucose and normalizes bowel regularity. This kind of action comes from a synergistic combination of flax, slippery elm, dulse, kelp seaweed, and North America-grown, organic psyllium in a low-carbohydrate meal replacement product called *Beyond Greens*, and in a healthy snack and fiber product called the Wholesome Fast Food (Fiber) Blend.

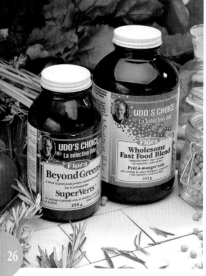

Beyond Greens and Wholesome Fast Food Blend

Healing Oils and the Immune System

Healing oils protect our genetic material (DNA) from damage. N-3 has anti-oxidant-like functions in the oil-soluble system of the body that is similar to the anti-oxidant function provided by vitamin C in a water-soluble system. Both protect you from damage because they are chemically active, and sacrifice themselves to substances that would otherwise damage vital structures in your cells.

Your immune system also uses healing fats to make oxygen bullets that it uses to kill infectious foreign invaders.

N-3 healing fats and derivatives of both n-3 and n-6 inhibit tumor growth.

Healing Oils and Candida

Healing oils help to reduce fungus infections like athlete's foot and yeast overgrowth or candida. The good fats kill these nasty

26

microorganisms quite effectively. Sometimes the yeast die-off is so rapid that it makes you feel like you have fog in your brain. This fog usually clears within a few weeks, when the liver has done its job of cleaning up and removing the yeast toxins from the body. Liver support and fiber help to speed up the detox process. Digestive enzymes reduce the load on digestive processes, thereby easing the liver's load.

Healing Oils and Osteoporosis

Healing oils are required for mineral transport and mineral metabolism. They keep bones strong, prevent bone mineral loss (osteoporosis and osteomalacia), and work against the tendency of protein metabolism to encourage bone mineral loss leading to brittle bones.

Research has shown that n-3 are especially effective at helping to deposit minerals in bones, and to prevent their loss from the bones and from the body.

Balancing Healing Oils with Protein

Healing oils are required for protein metabolism. Without them, proteins can become quite toxic. This was first shown in an animal study done in the early 1900's. Researchers starved dogs for several weeks and then fed them protein alone. The animals died quicker than if they had been fed nothing at all. In other words, the protein was toxic to the starved dogs. But when they gave the same protein along with essential fats, the dogs recovered very quickly from starvation.

People on high protein, or muscle-building, and low-fat or fat-phobic diets can induce serious health problems. In the absence of healing oils, protein can damage the liver, kidneys, and other inner organs.

Soothing the Digestive System with Healing Oils

Within our digestive tract, healing oils form a barrier against the absorption of undigested foods by improving gut integrity, slowing stomach emptying (allowing more time for digestion to take place), and by their anti-inflammatory effects. They help prevent leaky gut, a result of inflammation, and reduce food allergies.

Healing oils feed and protect friendly gut bacteria, and encourage the growth of beneficial bowel flora.

Healing oils help to greatly reduce the incidence of another

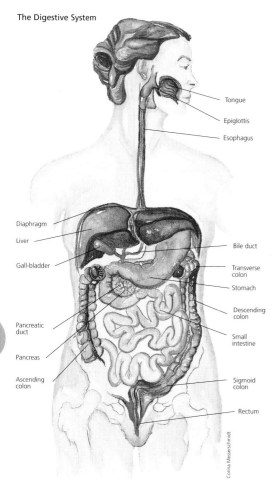

The Digestive System

Tongue
Epiglottis
Esophagus

Diaphragm
Liver
Gall-bladder

Bile duct
Transverse colon
Stomach
Descending colon
Small intestine

Pancreatic duct
Pancreas
Ascending colon

Sigmoid colon
Rectum

Corina Messerschmidt

common condition: constipation, and the toxic conditions that can result from a dehydrated colon, which is another way to describe constipation. Why do they help? By reducing the loss of water through the skin, they make it unnecessary for the body to pull water from the stool to replace the water lost through the skin, and so the stools stay softer.

Healing oils improve food flavors, because many flavors are oil-soluble. They also improve the absorption of oil-soluble phytonutrients that are poorly absorbed in their absence.

Skin as an indicator for establishing optimum intake

Healing oil plays an important role in the health of skin, hair, and nails. Dry skin is a clear indication that you're not getting enough oil in your diet. Use the feel of your skin to determine your optimum intake. Why? Because your skin gets the essential fats only after nature, in her wisdom, has provided them to your glands and inner organs with vital functions. Your skin gets them last and loses them first.

An optimum intake of healing oils contributes to soft, smooth, velvety skin without a hint of dryness. Oil forms a barrier against moisture loss. Applying them externally does not work as the oil may go rancid on your skin and then you could end up smelling like a fresh painting or furniture. Also, applying them to skin causes you to lose your best (dry skin) indicator for your optimum intake.

Most adults require between 2 and 5 tablespoons (30 and 75ml) of oil blend per day, mixed in foods. Some bodybuilders need 7 or 8 tablespoons (105 or 120 ml) to get the same feel I get on 3 or 4 tablespoons. The optimum depends on metabolic rate, activity level, body size, genetics, climate, season, and other factors.

We need more oil in winter than in summer. Weighing 175 pounds (80kg), I need about 3 tablespoons (45ml) per day in summer, but about 4 tablespoons (60ml) in winter. Flying from Vancouver to Denver in winter, I have noticed that my skin becomes dry within a few hours. A few extra tablespoons of the oil blend, and my skin is nice again within a few hours.

For eczema, acne, psoriasis, and other skin conditions, use healing oils in combination with digestive enzymes rich in protein-digesting protease enzymes. The oils improve gut integrity and decrease inflammation. Digestive enzymes ensure better digestion of foods. When foods are completely digested, allergies are less likely and symptoms are reduced.

Healing oils also prevent dehydration and problems caused by dehydration such as inflammation brought about by histamines and prostaglandin hormones.

Healing Oils and Detoxification

Healing oils can also be used for detoxification, when combined with a heat source such as a sauna. Oil-soluble toxins will leave the body in the oil part of the sweat. This was documented during the 1980's in a study on Agent Orange detoxification of Vietnam War veterans. They were put in a sauna for 15 to 30 minutes every day, for three to six months. The levels of Agent Orange were measured in the sweat, and the decrease in the body

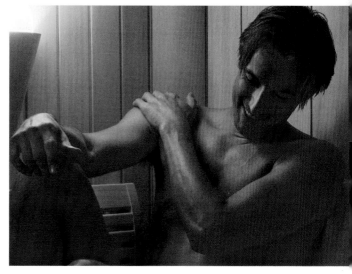

burden was monitored. Oils lost by sweating must be replaced to prevent dry skin. Healing oils best carry these toxins to the skin and out. Sweating can also remove DDT, PCBs, and other oil-soluble toxins from the body. Their removal through the skin is the safest exit route. Otherwise, liver or kidneys can be poisoned by these highly toxic, cancer-causing substances.

Recent research has also shown that n-3 fats can protect us from the toxic effects of pesticides in our tissues. Note: To prevent problems, be careful not to stay in the sauna too long. If you have cardiovascular problems, consult a knowledgeable health care professional.

For more information about the healing benefits of saunas read the book *Sauna - The Hottest Way to Good Health* by Giselle Roeder, an alive publication

Healing Oils and the Brain - Healing the Mind and Emotions

The brain needs healing oils to develop and function. It is the fat-richest organ in the body, with over 60% of the brain's dry weight composed of fats.

The ratio of n-3 to n-6 in the brain is 1: 1. The brain contains several other fats, and is rich in cholesterol. Lack of cholesterol can lead to impaired brain function. Healing oils can improve all areas of brain function: mood, intelligence, behavior, learning capacity, mental health, and socialization.

On diets providing optimum healing oil intake, many adults report feeling calmer. They deal with stress better. The healing oils are required for the production of serotonin, a neurotransmitter with calming effects. Many older people report better color perception and visual acuity; better mental processing and faster learning.

The essential fats found in healing oils are especially useful in three

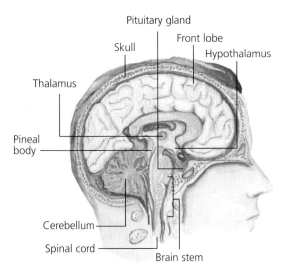

Pituitary gland
Skull
Front lobe
Hypothalamus
Thalamus
Pineal body
Cerebellum
Spinal cord
Brain stem

problem areas of brain function: learning problems; criminal behavior; and mental illness.

Brain development

Several recent studies point out the importance of healing oils for *pregnant women and children.* They show that the unborn child draws from its mother the essential n-3 and n-6 fats it needs for brain development. With each child, the mother becomes more depleted, and each child gets less healing oils from mother than the previous child.

When should a child begin to get healing oils? Three years before birth is ideal! Deficiencies in the mother can have a detrimental effect on children for up to 3 years after they are corrected. A pregnant woman needs to have enough healing oils for herself and her growing child. Nursing mothers need plenty of the healing oils in their diet, as her infant will draw 11g, almost half of an ounce, of essential fats from mother's breast milk each day. If you feed your baby formula or solid foods, add healing oils, as well as digestive enzymes and friendly bowel bacteria, since these are not present in formulas and commercial baby foods. They are important for the child's good health and development.

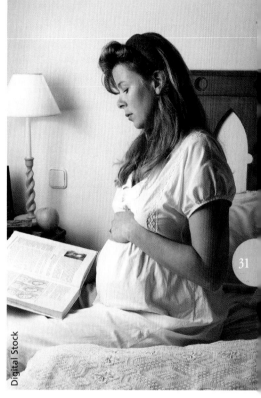

Digital Stock

31

Essential n-3 and n-6 fats are important for the unborn child's brain development

Researchers also suggest that depletion of healing oils explains why women have higher rates than men of depression, fibromyalgia, chronic fatigue, collagen diseases, inflammatory, and autoimmune conditions. Digestion problems and allergies should probably be added to that list. Women get these conditions from 2 to 9 times more frequently than men, and healing oil depletion during childbearing sets them up for all of these conditions.

Healing Mental Illness

Healing oils elevate mood and lift depression. Depressed children and adults benefit by improving their intake and balance of healing oils. Schizophrenics hallucinate less when their n-6 and especially n-3 intake is improved. Autism, Alzheimer's, and senility often respond well to healing oils.

Preliminary research suggests that healing oils will be useful in bipolar (or manic-depressive) as well as obsessive-compulsive disorder.

Recommended Optimum of Udo's Choice Oil Blend for People and Animals

PEOPLE: 30 – 75 ml per 100 pounds (45kg) of body weight per day

HORSES: 20 – 120 ml per 1,000 pounds (450kg) of body weight per day

DOGS: 0.5 – 2 ml per 10 pounds (4.5kg) per day

CATS: 0.5 –2 ml per 10 pounds (4.5kg) per day

The higher doses are used to obtain quicker results in situations of serious essential fats deficiency at the beginning of supplementation. Higher doses are also used for faster improved performance.

The figures above are general guidelines only, and individual animals differ somewhat in their optimum dosage. Guardians of animals should monitor their intake by the condition of their skin and coat. Optimum intake of healing oils produce full, shiny, beautiful fur, the animal equivalent of soft, velvety skin in humans. You will begin to see improvement within a month or less. Fully improved coat conditions may take up to 90 days at an optimum intake.

The 2: 1 ratio of n-3: n-6 that I recommend for people also works best for animals, for the same reason. Animal food tends to have the same n-3 deficiencies as do human foods.

Healing Fats Benefit Animals . . . .

Animals fed blended healing oils and oil seed products have healthier skin, hair, feathers, nails, and hooves. I have received positive feedback from owners of dogs, cats, hamsters, gerbils, rats, mice, horses, wild cats, elephants, wolves, hyenas, zebras, monkeys, and birds.

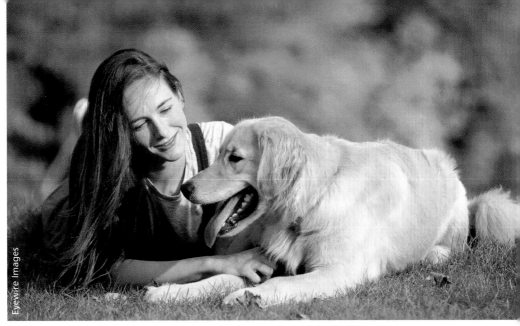

Improvement in skin conditions in dogs and cats, including dry skin, dandruff, skin inflammation, and hair loss are really obvious in 30 days. Horses develop a slick hair coat within a month. There is improvement even in show animals, already in top condition, within about two months.

Ensure the health of your dog through oil supplementation

Fleabites in dogs heal more rapidly. The fleas don't stop biting, but the bites swell less, the dogs don't scratch as much, and the healing is quicker. Healing oils speed skin repair.

Healing oils also speed healing from injuries and surgery.

By improving healing oil intake, hyperactive, nervous, skittish, horses can be calmed without behavior modification. Behavior in nervous dogs and cats also improves by adjusting their intake of the right fats to a level and ratio they would have obtained under ideal conditions in nature. Dogs and cats may not need as high an n-3: n-6 ratio as horses, but their natural diet contained both of these essential fats. Most commercial dog and cat foods contain no n-3, and less than optimum n-6.

Commercial animal foods are produced for shelf stability, convenience, and profit. N-3 is not even listed in the food manufacturing guidelines for dogs, cats, and horses. They are, however, known to be essential for monkeys. Their absence from pet food and livestock feed guidelines is, unfortunately, assurance that they will not be present in most animal foods.

In nature, horses live on a diet of greens that contain only about 0.1% fat. Eating 50 pounds of grass, an 1,100 pound horse might get about 25 grams (28ml or 2 tablespoons, close to one ounce) of healing oil per day. Optimum amount is higher than that. Horses in captivity can be fed to produce a much higher quality hair coat than wild horses normally have.

Dogs and cats need more fat than horses, but less than people. Cats require about the same amount per body weight as dogs.

Formula for Improving Animal Health

Udo's Choice Oil Blend is 100% oil, and gives quicker results than whole food products which are just under 20% oil, but the whole foods products contain a wider range of other nutrients beneficial for health. I recommend using both products for animals as well as their owners.

I use several whole food products for animals including Beyond Greens (n-3: n-6 ratio of 1.1: 1), and Wholesome Fast Food Blend (ratio of 1.7: 1). These products were developed for

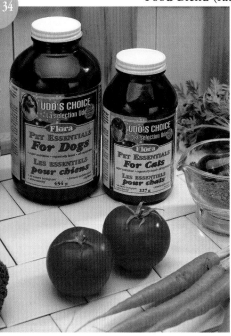

human consumption from mainly organically grown ingredients. But they also help improve health of companion animals. Beyond Greens emphasizes green foods, while Wholesome Fast Food Blend emphasizes fiber. For best results, feed animals about four times as much of the whole food product of oil blend.

You can also use products specifically developed for animals, containing organically based whole foods, food concentrates, vegetables, herbs, and extracts. We named the animal products PetEssentials for Dogs, PetEssentials for Cats, and HorsEssentials (n-3: n-6 ratio of about 1.8: 1).

All these products provide greens, fiber, and healing oils, which are in short supply in processed commercial animal foods. They enrich the diet of animals with major minerals, trace minerals, vitamins, soluble fiber, insoluble fiber, bowel flora, proteins, phytonutrients, and antioxidants from whole, natural foods, concentrates, and extracts. Plant-based enzymes are added to help with digestion. Herbs that support inner organ function are also included.

Add 1/3 to 8 tablespoons (5 to 120ml) per day of whole food products to the regular food of adult dogs (depending on the animal's weight). Use 1/5 to 2 teaspoons (1-10ml) for adult cats, and 1/2 to 3 cups (1/4 to 1.5 lbs.) per day for adult horses.

From Horsemeat to Champion

Let me tell you a story about a horse. In July 1999, a champion horse in Sweden, Emma by name, got kicked in the head by another horse. Her lower jaw was broken in several places. It was wired back together, but would not heal. The horse had open infected wounds and looked terrible. She stopped eating and drinking. Veterinarians worked on her for several months, and then gave up. They suggested to the owners that they turn this champion into horsemeat.

At this time, Emma's owner met a colleague of mine, and asked if she could help. She said she'd try. Unfortunately she was out of the Oil Blend at the time. But she did have some digestive enzymes. She gave the fallen champion two capsules, three times over the course of the day - six capsules in total. Within 24 hours, the inflammation had stopped. Then the healing oil blend arrived, and she started to feed oil to Emma. Within 6 days, the wound had been reduced from the size of a hand (20cm) to about 8cm across. The demeanor of the horse completely changed—from fearful and in pain—to tranquil. Then Emma was started on a mixture of 5 friendly gut bacteria (Super 5) to replace those killed by the vet's ineffective and damaging antibiotic treatments. She was also given Beyond Greens (a food replacement containing greens, fiber, protein, fats, herbs, enzymes, and antioxidants) and Wholesome Fast Food Blend, a product high in bowel-soothing mucilage fiber.

Emma's wound was completely healed in six weeks. A year later, Emma came 8th out of 150 horses in one of the most strenuous of equestrian events, the military chase.

There is an interesting additional finding that comes from this story. Emma had been given a lot of flax, because flax is known for improving skin and energy in horses. But it is less well known that flax can produce an n-6 deficiency because it has so much n-3 and so little n-6. This was my first experience with a horse becoming n-6 deficient on too much flax. I had previously observed this problem created by flax in many people and a few dogs.

Most domestic horses are fed corn oil, which gives them lots of n-6, but makes them n-3 deficient. N-3 deficiency symptoms include weakness, behavioral problems, and poor performance.

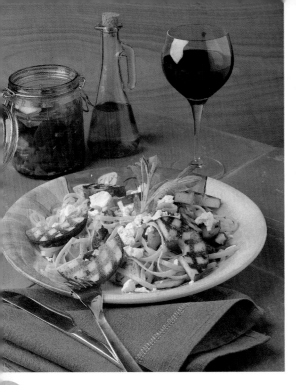

Integrate Essential Fats Into Your Diet . . . .

Healing Oils are Compatible with Many Foods.

Healing oils can be added to cold, warm, or hot dishes such as soup or steamed vegetables, but they should never be used for high temperature frying. Heating oil damages the essential fats, which then damage you.

Find cooking methods that are alternatives to frying, sautéing, and especially...deep fat frying. Poach, boil, steam, pressure cook, or eat foods raw, instead. Research done over the past 30 years has found a correlation between consuming fried fats and cancer, as well as hardening of the arteries.

Enjoy extra virgin olive oil the traditional Mediterranean way—drizzled fresh on pasta and salads, or steamed vegetables. Dip crusty bread in a mixture of oil, crushed garlic, and herbs. Avoid using olive oil as a medium for frying. Modern research has found that although olive oil has breast cancer-protective properties, they are lost when the oil is used to fry foods.

Drizzle healing oils on food to enhance the taste. Food flavor molecules are oil-soluble and the oil brings out the taste of, even, bland potatoes or breakfast oatmeal.

Yogurt and Kefir

Some athletes add the healing oil blend to their yogurt or protein shakes to get the necessary balance of proteins and fats, and then add a banana and other carbohydrate fuels they need for high performance. For breakfast, you can mix yogurt, greens, enzymes, probiotics, oil blend, and water together to make a shake. It tastes good. It's filling. And it's nutritious. You can also mix my healing oil blend with cottage cheese and other soft and hard cheeses or stir it into the yolk of soft-boiled eggs. Many health bars use the healing oil blend in juices and health drinks.

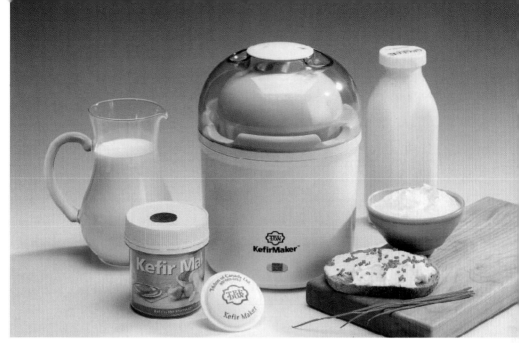

As an alternative to yogurt, good-tasting healthy, protein-rich kefir can be made from milk at home using a special Kefir Maker sold by a company called Teldon. I have tasted this kefir and can vouch for its delectable taste.

Essential fatty acids of the oil blend and lactic acids of kefir make an ideal combination.

37

Salads, Soups, Vegetables

The healing oil blend can be combined into any salad dressing. People who don't like vinegar use the oil blend by itself. Add it to soups after serving to the table. Use the oil blend on steamed vegetables, both to enhance flavors and to improve the absorption of the oil-soluble, health-enhancing phytonutrients in the vegetables. Make a dip using oil, spices, balsamic vinegar, yogurt and other ingredients. As a bonus, it makes raw vegetables less gassy.

Starches

Healing oils can be mixed into mashed potatoes or poured on baked ones, and are also wonderful on baked yams. Pour them on corn instead of butter. Be careful, though. These starchy foods will taste so good that you may eat them for pure pleasure, consume too much, and then the starch (not the healing oil!) will fatten you.

Juices

The healing oil blend can be added to nutritious fresh juices. It enhances the flavor and gives the juice more body. Adding healing oil to fruit juice is an easy way to integrate the right fats into your diet. The oil flavor is lost in the juice; the oil enhances the flavor of the juice; and the juice becomes more full-bodied.

Use fragrant juices such as: mango, peach, nectarine, pineapple, and tropical drinks. Or try apple, pear, grape, cherry, and orange juice. Or mix healing oils in applesauce!

Delicious oil combinations

Combine the healing oil blend in a food processor in a ratio of 50: 50 with butter or olive oil. It makes a lighter, more healthful product. Since butter and olive oil are poor sources of essential fats but have other virtues, the oil blend improves the nutritional profile and the health value of both. Extra virgin (green) olive oil is, in reality, a poor source of essential fats. 88% of the oil is made up of mono-unsaturated and saturated fatty acids that are not essential to your health because your body can manufacture them from sugar or starch. Olive oil contains only 10% n-6, and less than 1% n-3. But this traditional oil has a healthy reputation, based on the fact that it has not been over-processed, and still contains its phytonutrients. These benefit liver, gall bladder, digestive, immune, and cardio-vascular functions. Much of the health value of '100%' or 'extra light' olive oil, however, has been lost to processing.

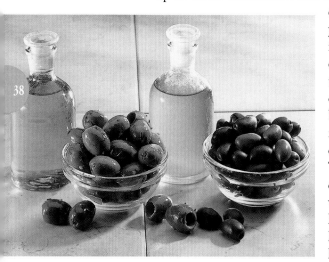

Unprocessed extra virgin olive oil contains phytonutrients not found in processed or refined oil

Healing oils allow you to enjoy saturated fats

Incorporate healing oils into your diet and you will also be able to eat saturated fats in moderation. Found in pork, beef, lamb, dairy foods, tropical nuts and seeds, they are natural and delicious and the body knows how to use them. They serve as fuel, and are a normal part of cell membrane structure. Saturated fats cause you health problems only when you eat too much of them while getting too few essential fats.

How much is safe? If you work as hard physically as your grandparents did, you can burn a lot of hard fats to produce the energy you need to do the strenuous work. Modern, more sedentary people need far less fuel.

Optimizing your intake of essential fats opens the door for you to use moderate amount of fresh, organic butter that is free of pesticides, antibiotics, and hormones. It allows you to put sour cream on your potatoes. But avoid margarine, because it is over-processed and not good for you.

Problems Introducing Healing Oils into your Diet

Are there limits to how much healing oil you can ingest? Symptoms of excessive intake can drowsiness, include and stomach upset. Too much oil on an empty stomach can cause nausea, the liver is reaction to over indulgence. It is better to add healing oils to food, and to spread your intake out over the course of the day.

Sleeplessness

If you take essential fat-rich oils too close to bedtime, you may not be able to sleep because they will increase your energy level. It is best not to take essential fat-rich oils after 8:00 p.m. Taken earlier essential fats improve the quality of sleep.

Stomach upsets

If you ingest more healing oils than your liver can handle at any one time, you may feel full, heavy, or nauseous. The amount the liver can handle differs with individuals. I have taken up to 15 tablespoons over the course of a day. Once, I took 17 tablespoons for breakfast, mixed with tropical fruit juice. I discovered my limit. I wasn't hungry the rest of the day. If I had taken 20 tablespoons, I probably would have felt sick to my stomach.

Some people have problems taking just one or two tablespoons. It's an indication of limited liver function or liver toxicity overload. If this happens to you, reduce the amount you use at any one time, spread the servings out over the course of the day, and mix the oil with foods. Start with a small amount, and gradually increase it. Negotiate a balance that works for you. Take as much as you can handle. If you cannot handle three tablespoons, use one. If one is too much, use a teaspoon. If that's too much, take a few drops. If you can't handle that, take a lick. And if a lick's too much, take a whiff. But don't quit, because every cell in your body requires healing oils and their essential fats.

Some people used to low fat or fat free diets have weak liver function, and are repelled by the smell or sight of oil. They have to start small, and can gradually increase their dose as their liver regains its function. If you have this problem, try a little oil mixed with apple sauce or fruit juice. It will cut the oil and help you overcome your aversion to fat.

Occasionally, someone has an allergic response to oil. Then it should be taken with digestive enzymes. If this does not work, find another source of essential fats. Allergy to oil is rare, even in individuals sensitive to the seeds and nuts from which the oils are pressed. This is because proteins trigger most allergies, and oils are generally protein-free. In fact, the essential fat-rich oils usually help to relieve allergy symptoms.

Product Information - Whole food products developed by the author . . . .

Beyond Greens, Wholesome Fast Food Blend, PetEssentials for Dogs, PetEssentials for Cats, and *HorsEssentials* provide fiber, protein, essential fats, amino acids, major minerals, trace minerals, vitamins, anti-oxidants, enzymes, and friendly bacteria.

Udo's Choice Oil Blend provides a concentrated source of healing essential fats, and makes it convenient to obtain optimum intake of the essential fats for humans, as well as animals. The oil is produced by methods developed by the author between 1983 and 1986 for making oils with health (rather than shelf life) in mind. Use one to four tablespoons per day of the oil blend in addition to *Beyond Greens* or *Wholesome Fast Food Blend.* Flora, Inc., Flora Manufacturing and Distributing, and FMD produce the oil blend and other products. They are available in health food stores in Canada, the US, Australia, and Europe, and from health practitioners, trainers, sports nutrition stores and gyms in North America, Europe, and Australia.

Digestive Enzyme Blend, and *Super 5 Probiotics* have been developed by the author to improve health by improving digestion and ensuring the presence of friendly microorganisms in the gut.

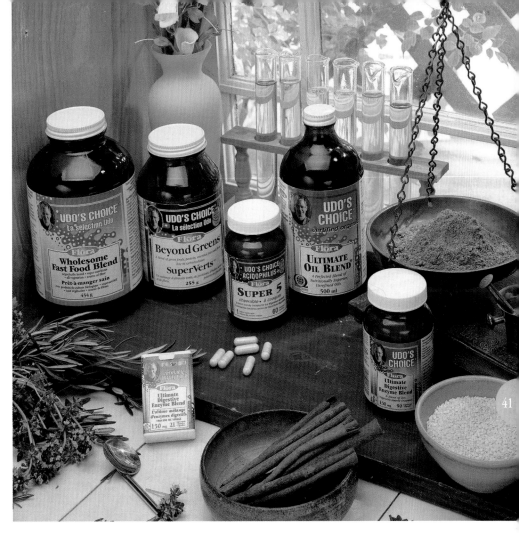

Udo's Choice Health Plan for the new millennium is an audiotape (no charge) about these products including their background, target, manufacture, use, and storage. There is also a brochure by the same name, which describes the products in a different way, and an 8-page report called *Perfected Health Plan for the New Millennium.* These are available through health food stores in North America and through international distributors.

The Perfected Health Plan audiotape and further information is available, free of charge, from retail stores or by calling 1-800-446-2110 in the US; 1-800-663-0617 in Canada, and through international distributors.

The finest raw ingredients are required for high quality nutritional products.

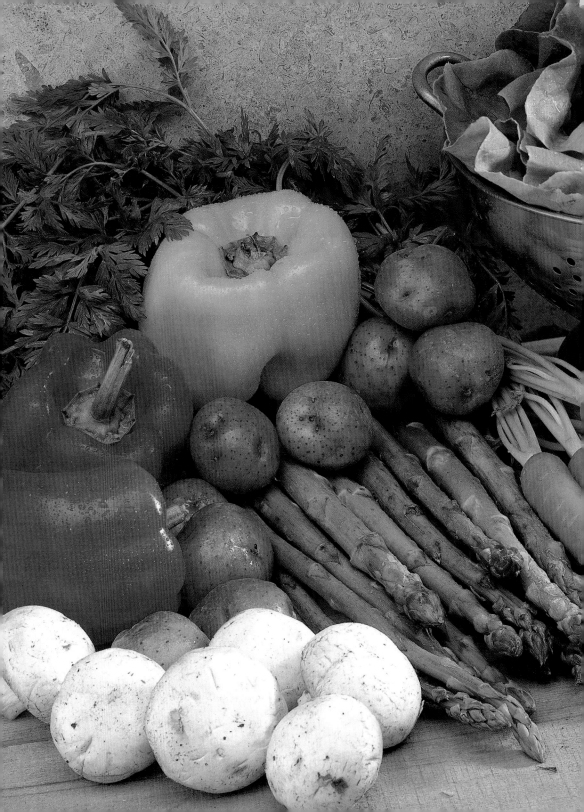

Learn how to use healing fats
and oils in your healthful meals

Marinated Goat Cheese with Mediterranean Spices

Like a good book, you can take this marinated cheese everywhere with you—it greatly enhances a summer's salad and is perfect for picnics. The oil-and-spice marinade boosts the flavor of goat or feta cheese. Simply use it in wraps and on pizzas. I recommend tossing it in your salad with some of its oil and a bit of lemon juice.

1½ cups (300 g) goat cheese or (450 g) feta cheese, cubed

2 dry limes, pierced with knife, or 2 slices lemon

1 tsp (5 mL) fennel seed

1 tsp (5 mL) mustard seed

1-2 pieces star anise

2 bay leaves

5-6 juniper berries

2-3 pieces cloves

3-4 cloves garlic

1½ cups (375 mL) Udo's oil

In a 2-cup (500-mL) airtight glass jar, layer the cheese, dry lime (or lemon slices) and spices. Fill with oil and refrigerate. Use a clean fork to take out some cheese to prevent bacteria from entering the container, and keep lid tightly closed. Cheese marinated this way keeps 2 to 3 months in the refrigerator, although it tastes so wonderful, it won't last for more than a few weeks.

Variations: Make sure you try both hard and soft types of goat cheese. I recommend the ones with herbs added. Cut hard cheeses in cubes and soft ones in slices then cover with oil.

Kitchen Tips for Healthy Oils

It is always best to eat oils in their natural, unheated form. Healthy unrefined oils add flavor and nutrition when mixed in salad dressings and dips, and drizzled over soups and stirred in cooked dishes.

Never fry these oils: flaxseed, walnut, soybean, Udo's oil blend, other EFA-rich blends, pumpkinseed, safflower and sunflower oil. For light sautéing, butter or coconut oil are the most suitable, as long as their temperatures are kept below smoke point. These oils are less damaged in frying than liquid oils, and therefore result in less toxicity. Steamed, poached, boiled, pressure-cooked or raw foods are better for health.

Extra-virgin olive oil is not recommended for frying if health is important to you. Surprised? Traditionally, food was prepared using water, then drizzled with olive oil once it was off the stove. Olive oil is a surprisingly delicate, easily damaged oil.

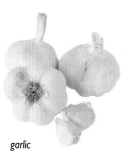

garlic

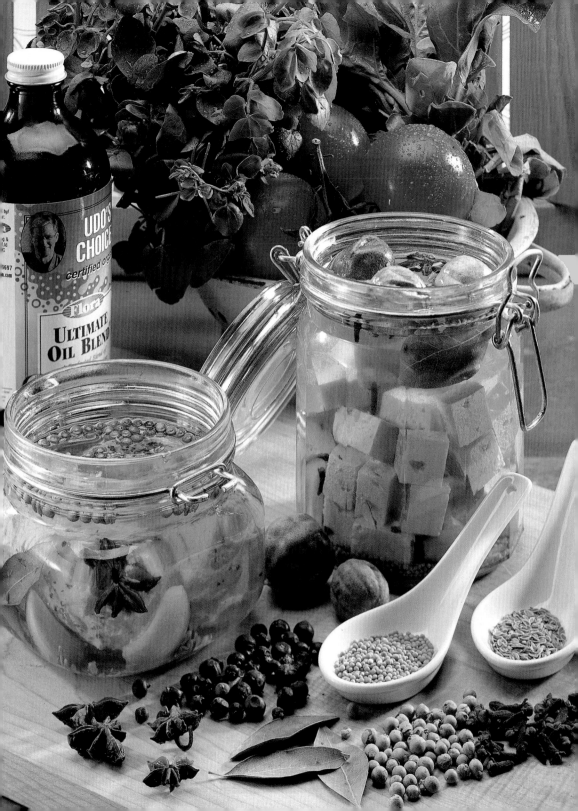

Sunny Feta Oil Salad

The heart of the romaine tastes sweet but don't forgo the extra nutrition in the darker outer leaves. The combination of vegetables and herbs enhanced with Udo's oil evokes the fresh taste of summer.

¼ cup (60 mL) Udo's oil

2 tbsp (30 mL) fresh lemon juice

1 tsp (5 mL) fresh oregano, chopped

1 tsp (5 mL) fresh basil, chopped

1 tsp (5 mL) fresh parsley, chopped

2 cups (500 mL) romaine lettuce

1 cup (250 mL) cherry tomatoes, cut in half

1 cup (250 mL) cucumber, cut in chunks

1 cup (250 mL) each red and yellow bell peppers, cut in chunks

1 cup (250 mL) red onion, sliced

1 cup (250 mL) marinated goat or feta cheese (see page ?)

½ cup (125 mL) kalamata or green olives

Vegetable salt, to taste

In a large bowl, combine oil, lemon juice, oregano, basil and parsley. Add lettuce, tomato, cucumber, peppers, onion, cheese and olives; toss well. Season to taste and serve.

Serves 4

Cut romaine lettuce only when you're ready to use it, because the ends oxidize quickly. Discard outermost leaves if brown or damaged, wash remainder carefully then soak in filtered water for 20 minutes. Wrap in clean paper towels, place in a plastic bag and refrigerate for up to six days.

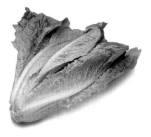

Romaine lettuce

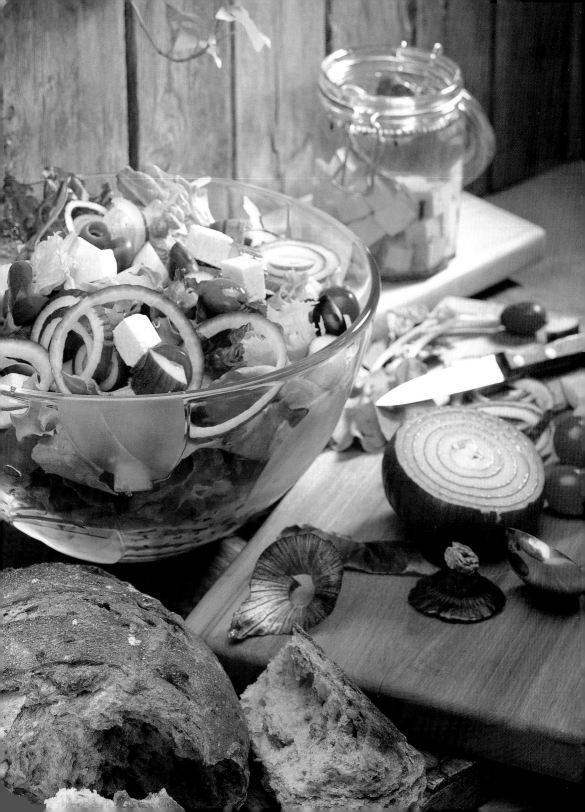

Frisée Salad with Lemon-Thyme Vinaigrette

Frisée lettuce, also called curly endive, gives any salad extra zing. Its slightly bitter flavor makes it a wonderful food for detoxifying your liver. Udo's oil combined with lemon juice, vinegar and herbs adds a wonderful aroma and a healthy touch to complete your cleansing experience.

4 cups (1 L) frisée lettuce

½ cup (125 mL) carrot, balled or cubed

½ cup (125 mL) kohlrabi, balled or cubed

½ cup (125 mL) zucchini, balled or cubed

½ cup (125 mL) bell pepper, diced

½ cup (125 mL) cherry tomatoes

Lemon-Thyme Vinaigrette:

½ cup (125 mL) Udo's oil

¼ cup (60 mL) lemon juice

1 tsp (5 mL) apple cider vinegar

1 tsp (5 mL) Dijon mustard

Vegetable salt, to taste

1½ tbsp (25 mL) shallot or onion, minced

1 tbsp (15 mL) red or yellow bell pepper, finely diced

1 tbsp (15 mL) chives or green onion, chopped

1 tsp (5 mL) fresh thyme

To make the vinaigrette, blend oil, lemon juice, vinegar, mustard and seasoning with a whisk or hand blender to emulsify. Stir in shallot, pepper, chives and thyme.

Toss with vegetables and serve. Save any remaining vinaigrette in the refrigerator for up to one week.

Serves 4

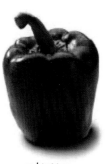

red pepper

Curly endive belongs to the chicory family and is a good source of vitamins A and C, calcium and magnesium. Look for endive with crisp leaves. Refrigerate in the crisper and use within five days.

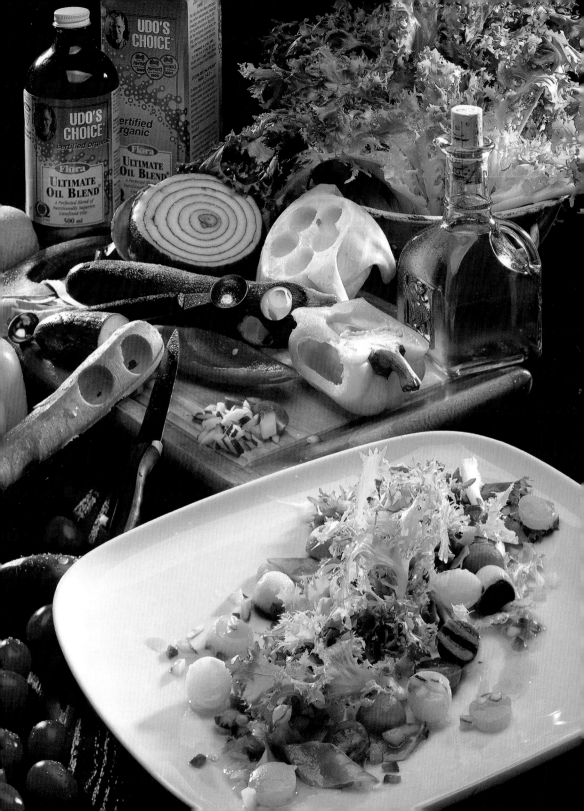

Corn Tortillas with Salsa and Guacamole

Adding healthy oils immediately improves the nutrition profile of these classic party pleasers. Tomatoes are excellent sources of vitamin C and good sources of vitamins A, B complex, E, folate and fiber. Oil enhances the absorption of the tomato's lycopene, which has antioxidant, anticancer, and prostate-protective properties. Avocados are a highly nourishing food, being rich in valuable fats.

Salsa:

2 cups (500 mL) tomato, finely diced

1 cup (250 mL) black beans, cooked

½ cup (125 mL) onion, finely diced

¼ cup (60 mL) each green, red and yellow peppers, finely diced

2 tbsp (30 mL) fresh mint or cilantro, chopped

3 cloves garlic, minced

¼ cup (60 mL) Udo's oil

2 tbsp (30 mL) fresh squeezed lemon juice

Guacamole:

4 ripe avocados

2 tbsp (30 mL) fresh cilantro, chopped

¼ cup (60 mL) onion, finely diced

½ cup (125 mL) tomato, finely diced

½ cup (125 mL) sour cream, yogurt or kefir

¼ cup (60 mL) Udo's oil

2 tbsp (30 mL) fresh squeezed lemon juice

Sea salt or vegetable salt, to taste

To make the salsa, combine the ingredients in a bowl and refrigerate for 2 hours before serving, in order for the flavors to incorporate. Raw tomatoes are best served at room temperature for maximum flavor.

To make the guacamole, mash avocado in a bowl, leaving some chunks, and combine with remaining ingredients. Serve at room temperature or slightly chilled.

Serve both salsa and guacamole with organic corn tortilla chips.

Variation: Add fresh corn kernels to the salsa when they're in season.

Serves 4

Local, seasonal vine-ripened tomatoes have the best flavor and the most vitamin C. Ripe tomatoes keep up to ten days refrigerated uncovered in the crisper.

Choose avocados that are heavy for their size. They're ready to eat when they yield slightly when gently squeezed. Store at room temperature until ripe, then refrigerate until ready to use.

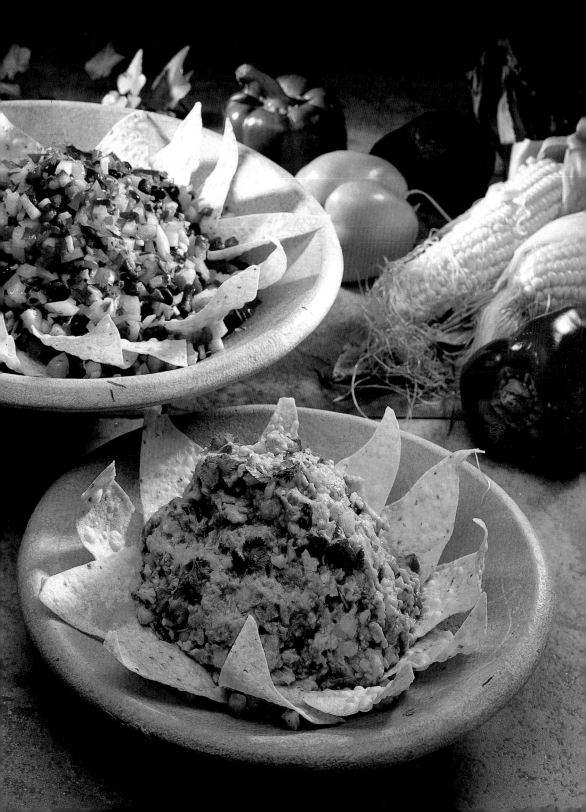

Minestrone with Parmesan Croutons

This delicious hearty soup makes an ideal luncheon, with enough high-quality protein, carbohydrates, vitamins, minerals and essential fats to give you energy to run a marathon.

1 cup (250 mL) eggplant, cubed

1 cup (250 mL) nugget potato, cubed

1 cup (250 mL) zucchini, cubed

1 cup (250 mL) carrots, diced

½ cup (125 mL) onion, chopped

2 cloves garlic, minced

2 tbsp (30 mL) coconut oil

1 cup (250 mL) navy beans, cooked

1 cup (250 mL) green beans, cut 1" (3 cm) and blanched

2 cups (500 mL) vegetable stock or filtered water

2 cups (500 mL) tomato juice

Sea salt or vegetable salt, to taste

4 slices whole wheat baguette

2 tbsp (30 mL) butter

Parmesan cheese, freshly grated

In a large pot, gently sauté eggplant, potato, zucchini, carrot, onion and garlic in coconut oil for 2 to 3 minutes. Add navy beans, vegetable stock and tomato juice; bring to a boil and simmer for 10 to 12 minutes. Season to taste.

In the meantime, blanch green beans in boiling salted water for 4 minutes. Drain and rinse with cold water.

To make the croutons, spread both sides of bread with butter then place under the broiler for 2 to 3 minutes until golden.

Spoon soup into bowls then add green beans and drizzle with Udo's oil. Place crouton on top of the soup and top with freshly grated Parmesan cheese.

Serves 4

Blanch green beans and add them at the end of cooking because tomato juice contains acid that oxidizes and turns the beans brown. If the color of the beans doesn't bother you, you can cook them with the rest of the vegetables.

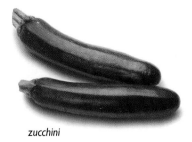

zucchini

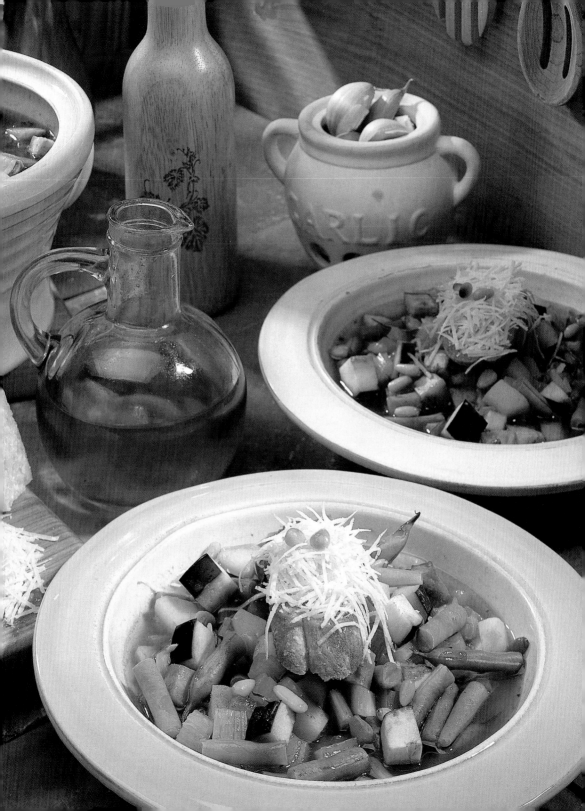

Traditional Tofu Soup with Oriental Vegetables

Asian cultures are famous for making simple and easy dishes. Traditional vegetable soup warms the home, brings the family together and keeps the spirit strong, the body healthy and the mind wise.

4 cups (1 L) vegetable stock or filtered water

1 cup (250 mL) baby corn

1 cup (250 mL) daikon, julienned

½ cup (125 mL) baby carrots, julienned

½ cup (125 mL) each red and yellow bell pepper, julienned

½ cup (125 mL) celery, sliced diagonally

¼ cup (60 mL) green peas

Small bunch baby bok choy, cut in half lengthwise

1½ cups (375 mL) organic firm tofu, cubed

½ cup (125 mL) organic soybean sprouts

¼ cup (60 mL) green onion, chopped

4 tbsp (60 mL) Udo's oil

4 slices lime, for garnish

In a large pot, bring vegetable stock (or filtered water) to a boil. Add corn, daikon, carrots, peppers, celery, green peas, bok choy and tofu; simmer for 5 to 7 minutes. Stir in sprouts and green onion then pour into bowls. Drizzle with oil, garnish with lime and serve.

Serves 4

The proper storage of healthy oils

When mixing and storing oils in vinaigrettes, dressings or dips, use glass jars as the oil tends to take on the smell of plastic containers.

Keep oils away from light to avoid deterioration and from air to prevent oxidation. Brown glass bottles are best, then green, then clear, in that order. A box around the brown glass bottle excludes all light and is advised for the most sensitive oils.

Using the freshest oils tastes the best and gives you maximum nutrition. When buying, remember to check the "best before" date. When you bring the bottle home, open it and taste a bit of the oil. Memorize the fresh taste, then when you use it the next time, taste it again to see if it's still the same flavor. You'll know when an oil is spoiled. It will taste unpalatable, similar to cod liver and other fish oils, which usually have a high level of rancidity.

Oils can be frozen solid to extend shelf life. Oils shrink when they freeze, so the glass bottle will not break. Freezing retains oil freshness for two years or more. The shelf date on the label, based on keeping the oil refrigerated, can then be ignored.

Once opened, keep oil in the refrigerator and use up within three to twelve weeks depending on the oil, because it will start to go rancid on contact with air. It's important to buy oils in small quantities such as in 8 ounce or 16 ounce (250 mL or 500 mL) bottles to avoid wasting oil due to spoilage.

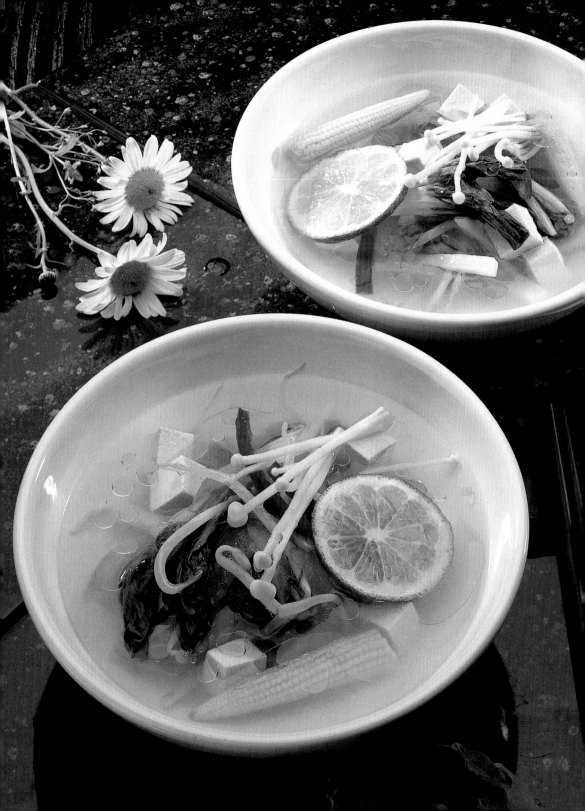

Spaghetti with Pesto Cashews and Asiago

The combination of basil pesto, cashew nuts and Asiago cheese enhances the simple spaghetti with unforgettable flavors and interesting textures. Served with a mild salad and cherry tomatoes, you'll have a nutritious meal that satisfies even the largest appetite.

14 oz (400 g) whole wheat spaghetti

¼ cup (60 mL) raw cashews

Freshly shaved Asiago cheese

Fresh basil, for garnish

Pesto:

½ cup (125 mL) pine nuts

3 lbs (1.3 kg) fresh basil leaves

1/4 cup (60 mL) garlic, chopped

1 cup (250 mL) Udo's oil

1 tbsp (15 mL) sea salt or vegetable salt

¼ cup (60 mL) Parmesan cheese, grated

To make the pesto, heat a cast-iron pan and gently warm pine nuts on low to intensify flavor. Wash and dry the basil thoroughly then place in a food processor with garlic and pine nuts. Blend and slowly add oil until a thick creamy sauce. Add seasoning and blend again. Stir in Parmesan (do not blend).

In a pan, warm cashews on low to intensify flavor. Cook pasta in a large pot of boiling salted water. Drain, rinse and toss immediately with 1/2 cup (125 mL) pesto and cashews. Do not heat pesto sauce, the pasta is hot enough to warm it.

Place pasta onto plates and sprinkle shaved Asiago over top. Garnish with fresh basil.

Variations: You can make a variety of pesto sauces. Try arugula, parsley, thyme, bell pepper or sun-dried tomatoes. Pesto keeps in the refrigerator for about one week or freeze it.

Roasting nuts on high heat destroys the good fats. Instead, gently heat nuts in a pan on low heat to intensify their flavor without burning them, and to enhance digestibility and destroy surface mold.

"Raw" cashews are technically not raw. The nut is encased in a shell that's toxic to the skin and causes blisters. Freshly picked cashews are roasted or dropped in boiling water to release the toxins before the nuts are extracted from their shells. Cashews are low in essential fats compared to other nuts, but high in protein, magnesium, phosphorus and potassium. Fresh cashews are crisp, white and sweet-tasting, and best bought whole rather than in pieces.

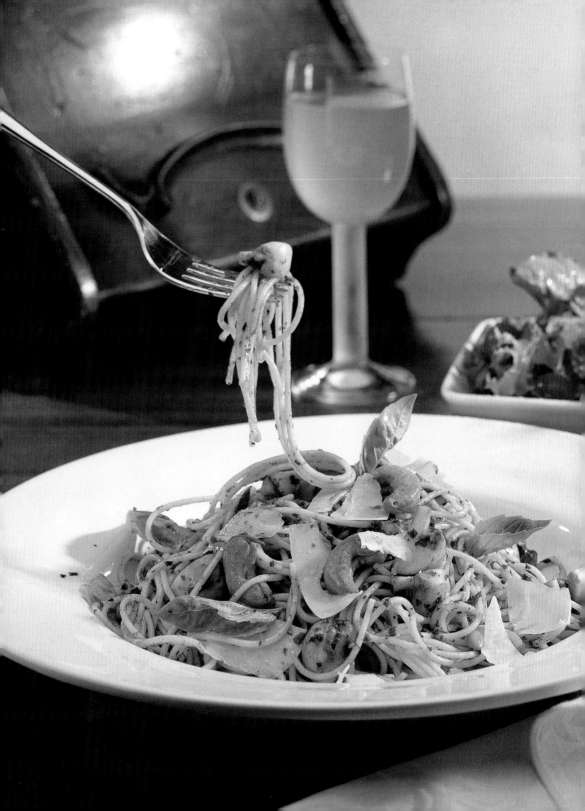

Tuna Fillet with Crispy Wonton Salad

The (blue fin) tuna is a very tasty high-protein, low-fat fish with a delicate, enjoyable texture.

4 tuna fillets (¼ lb/125 g each)

Pinch sea salt

Pinch wasabi powder (optional)

2 tbsp (30 mL) fresh squeezed lemon juice

Salad:

½ package wonton wrap, finely shredded

1 cup (250 mL) coconut oil

2 cups (500 mL) mixed organic greens

1 cup (250 mL) daikon radish or regular radish, finely shredded

1 tbsp (15 mL) each red and yellow bell pepper, finely chopped

1 tbsp (15 mL) red onion, finely chopped

1 tbsp (15 mL) green onion, chopped, for garnish

Thai Dressing:

1 tsp (5 mL) lemon grass, finely chopped

1 tbsp (15 mL) each red and yellow bell pepper, diced

1 tbsp (15 mL) shallot, minced

¼ cup (60 mL) sesame seed oil

¼ cup (60 mL) Udo's oil

2 tsp (10 mL) teriyaki sauce

2 tsp (10 mL) honey

1 tsp (5 mL) hoisin sauce

Pinch cracked chili, to taste

In a pan, heat coconut oil and cook wonton for 1 minute until crisp. Remove wonton from the pan and place on a paper towel to absorb excess oil.

Wash tuna and dry carefully with a paper towel. Sprinkle both sides with salt, wasabi (if desired) and lemon juice. In a separate pan, heat 2 tablespoons (30 mL) of the same coconut oil, and sear the tuna fillets for 1 1/2 to 2 minutes each side. Remove from pan and slice in 1/4" (5 mm) strips. The tuna will be slightly raw on the inside.

To make the dressing, blend together all dressing ingredients until emulsified. In a mixing bowl, combine greens, radish, peppers, red onion and wonton then toss with 1/4 cup (60 mL) of the dressing.

Place salad onto plates and arrange tuna slices around. Sprinkle with green onion and serve.

Serves 4

When choosing fresh fish, look for fish smelling only of salt water (no fishy smell), with a bright shiny color and tight muscles with no cracks in the filet.

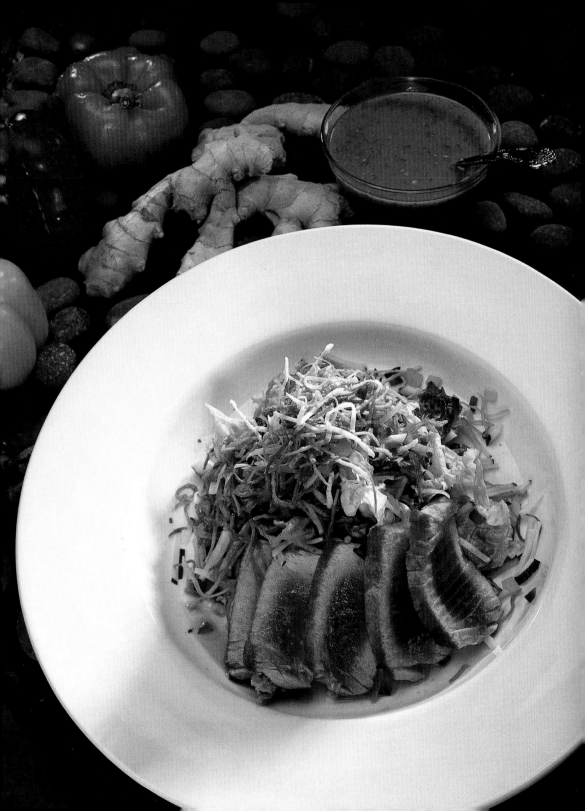

Sea Bass with Asian Dressing

The banana leaf imparts a nice woody taste to the delicate flavor of the sea bass. Buy the leaves fresh or dried (soak in water first) in Asian food stores. Together with the steamed vegetables, wild rice and healthful dressing, you'll have a meal that fully satisfies both stomach and taste buds.

4 sea bass fillets, (about ¼ lb/125 g each)

2 banana leaves

Vegetable salt, to taste

2 cups (500 mL) carrot, julienned

2 cups (500 mL) zucchini, julienned

2 cups (500 mL) daikon, julienned

2 tbsp green onion, chopped

Asian Dressing:

1 tbsp (15 mL) fresh cilantro, chopped

1 tbsp (15 mL) ginger, minced

1 tbsp (15 mL) garlic, minced

1 tsp (5 mL) tamari

1 tbsp (15 mL) fresh squeezed lemon juice

4 tbsp (60 mL) Udo's oil

1 tsp (5 mL) sesame seeds (optional)

Line a bamboo steamer with banana leaves then place sea bass on top. Season with vegetable salt then steam bass for 7 to 10 minutes depending on the thickness of the fillets. Cook carrot, zucchini, daikon and green onion in another bamboo steamer stacked on top of first steamer for 4 minutes (or blanch vegetables for 4 minutes in boiling salted water then drain and rinse with cold water).

In the meantime, combine dressing ingredients in a bowl. Place vegetables onto plates, arrange fish on top, and spoon dressing over top. Serve with wild brown rice (recipe in box).

Variation: Line the bamboo steamer with lemon grass for a different flavor.

Serves 4

> **Wild Brown Rice**
> Cook 2 cups (500 mL) of brown rice in 4 cups (1 L) filtered water until water is fully absorbed. Cook 1 cup (250 mL) of wild rice in 2 1/2 to 3 cups (625 to 750 mL) water. Mix rice together.

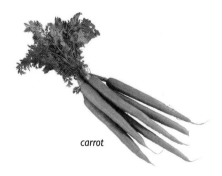

carrot

60

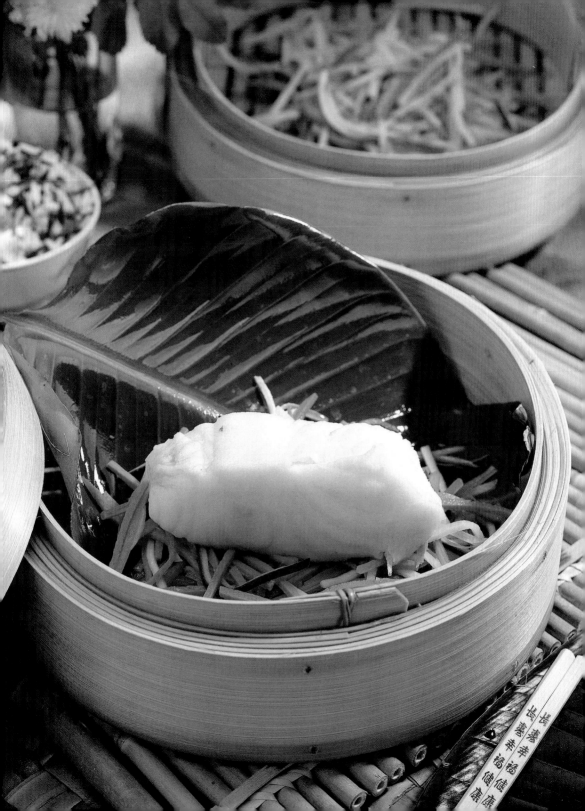

Books

The following books are excellent compilations of thousands of research studies, and contain hundreds of useful references that you can use to follow up on specific topics.

- Budwig J, Die elementare Funktion der Atmung in ihrer Beziehung zu autoxydablen Nahrungstoffen. Hyperion Verlag, Freiburg, Germany. 1953.
- Budwig J, Das Fettsyndrom (The Fat Syndrome). Hyperion Verlag, Freiburg, Germany. 1959.
- Crawford M & Marsh D, Nutrition and Evolution. Keats Publishing, New Canaan, CT. 1995.
- Erasmus U, Fats That Heal Fats That Kill. alive Books, Burnaby, Canada. 1993.
- Faigin R, Natural Hormone Enhancement: the Ultimate Strategy for Lifetime Youthfulness, Physical Transformation, and Super-Health. Extique Publishing, Cedar Mountain, NC. 2000. Chapter 18 contains a good summary of fats and fat-burning.
- Horrobin D, Omega-6 Essential Fatty Acids: Pathophysiology and Roles in Clinical Medicine. Wiley-Liss, NY, NY. 1990.
- Horrobin D, (ed) Clinical Uses of Essential Fatty Acids. Eden Press, Montreal, QU. 1982.
- Mudd C, Cholesterol and your health: the great American rip-off. American Lite Co, Oklahoma City, OK. 1990.
- Rudin DO & Felix C, Omega 3 Oils: to improve mental health, fight degenerative diseases, and extend your life. Avery Publishing Group, Garden City, NY. 1996.
- Simopoulos AP, The Omega Plan. Harper-Collins, NY, NY. 1998.
- Schmidt MA, Smart Fats: how dietary fats and oils affect mental, physical, and emotional intelligence. Frog, Ltd, Berkeley, CA. 1997.
- Wysong RL, Lipid Nutrition: understanding fats and oils in health and disease. Inquiry Press, Midland, MI. 1990.

Research Studies

Tens of thousands of studies on essential fats have been published. Look for them in libraries and the Internet. Below are a few that have been particularly interesting and helpful to me.

Ascherio A et al Trans Fatty Acid Intake and Risk of Myocardial Infarction. Circulation 1994; 89-94.

Ascherio A & Willett WC Health Effects of Trans Fatty Acids. American Journal of Clinical Nutrition 1997; 66(Suppl): 1006S-1010S.

Ascherio A et al Trans Fatty Acids and Coronary Heart Disease. New England Journal of Medicine 1999 Jun 24; 340(25): 1994-8.

Brunner R Dietary Fat and Ischemic Stroke. Journal of the American Medical Association 1998 Apr 15; 279 (15): 1171-2.

Caruso D et al Effect of Virgin Olive Oil Phenolic Compounds on In Vitro Oxidation of Human Low Density Lipoproteins. Nutrition and Metabolism in Cardiovascular Disease 1999 Jun; 9(3): 102-7.

Clarke Steven D Polyunsaturated fatty acid regulation of gene transcription: a mechanism to improve energy balance and insulin resistance. British Journal of Nutrition 2000; 83: Suppl. 1, S59-S66.

Crawford M et al Role of Plant-Derived Omega-3 Fatty Acids in Human Nutrition. Annals of Nutrition & Metabolism 2000; 44(5-6): 263-5.

Eritsland J Safety Considerations of Polyunsaturated Fatty Acids. American Journal of Clinical Nutrition 2000 Jan; 71(1 Suppl): 197S-201S.

Jump DR & Clarke SD Regulation of Gene Expression by Dietary Fat. Annual Review of Nutrition 1999; 19: 63-90.

Raheja BS et al Significance of the N-6/N-3 Ratio for Insulin Action in Diabetes. Annals of the New York Academy of Sciences 1993; 683: 258-71.

Ross JA et al The Anti-Catabolic Effects of N-3 Fatty Acids. Current Opinion in Clinical Nutrition and Metabolic Care 1999 May; 2(3): 219-26.

Simopoulos AP The Role of Fatty Acids in Gene Expressions: Health Implications. Annals of Nutrition & Metabolism 1996; 40: 303-311.

Simopoulos AP Essential Fatty Acids in Health and Chronic Disease. American Journal of Clinical Nutrition 1999 Sep; 70(3 Suppl): 560S-569S.

Simopoulos AP Human Requirement for N-3 Polyunsaturated Fatty Acids. Poultry Science 2000 Jul: 79(7): 961-70.